W9-AYC-881

Hyperactivity, The So-Called Attention-Deficit Disorder, And The Group of MBD Syndromes

Hyperactivity, The So-Called Attention-Deficit Disorder, And The Group of MBD Syndromes

RICHARD A. GARDNER, M.D.

Clinical Professor of Child Psychiatry,
Columbia University,
College of Physicians and Surgeons

Creative Therapeutics
155 County Road, Cresskill, New Jersey 07626-0317

© 1987 by Creative Therapeutics
155 County Road, Cresskill, New Jersey 07626-0317

PRINTED IN THE UNITED STATES OF AMERICA

10 9 8 7 6 5 4 3 2 1

Library of Congress Cataloging-in-Publication Data
Gardner, Richard A.
   Hyperactivity, the so-called attention-deficit
disorder, and the group of MBD syndromes.

   Bibliography: p.
   Includes index.
   1. Attention-deficit disorders.   2. Hyperactive child
syndrome.   I. Title.   [DNLM: 1. Attention-Deficit Disorder
with Hyperactivity.   WS 350.6 G228h]
RJ496.A86G37 1987   618.92'8589   87-13499
ISBN 0-933812-15-9

I dedicate this book to:

    Andrew Kevin
    Nancy Tara
    Julie Anne
    Tracy Mayle
    Katelijne Angelique
    and David

Other Books by Richard A. Gardner

All the world's a stage,
And all the men and women merely players:
They have their exits and their entrances;
And one man in his time plays many parts....

William Shakespeare

All the world's a bell-shaped curve,
And all the men and women merely numbers:
They have their means and their standard deviations;
And one man in his time appears on many curves....

Richard A. Gardner

Contents

Acknowledgments

I am indeed fortunate in having many accomplished friends and colleagues who have provided vital assistance in the preparation of this book. Their contributions were especially useful in areas in which I cannot claim expertise, e.g. pediatrics, statistics, and obstetrics-gynecology. Their valuable advice has, without question, added to the strength and value of the material presented and, I am sure, will protect me from embarrassment as well.

In the realm of pediatrics, I am grateful for the recommendations of Russell Asnes, M.D., Clinical Professor of Pediatrics, Columbia University, College of Physicians and Surgeons; Michael Katz, M.D., Professor and Chairman, Department of Pediatrics, Columbia University, College of Physicians and Surgeons; and Stanley Plotkin, M.D., Professor of Pediatrics, University of Pennsylvania. For their input into the experimental design and statistical analysis of the data I am indebted to my son Andrew K. Gardner, President of MEDCAL, an educational computer software company; Judith Green, Ph.D., Professor of Psychology, The William Paterson College of New Jersey; and Charles A. Opsahl, Ph.D., Assistant Professor of Psychology, Department of Psychiatry, Yale University School of Medicine. Valuable contributions in the field of obstetrics and gynecology were provided by Michael Weingarten, M.D., Associate Clinical Professor of Obstetrics and Gynecology, New Jersey College of Medicine and Dentistry.

The above individuals helped at the ideational level. At the more practical level I am deeply appreciative of the contributions of my secretaries Linda Gould, Carol Gibbon, and Donna La Tourette. As they have so many times in the past, they dedicated themselves enthusiastically to the typing of the manuscript in its various renditions. I am grateful to Mr. Robert Tebbenhoff for his valuable input into the production of this book, from manuscript to final volume.

My greatest debt, however, is to those children and families who have taught me much over the years about the neurologically based learning and behavioral difficulties described in this book. What I have learned from their sorrows and grief will, I hope, contribute to the prevention and alleviation of such unfortunate experiences by others.

Introduction

I use the term *Group of Minimal Brain Dysfunction Syndromes* as a rubric under which is subsumed a variety of neurologically based brain disorders, e.g. learning disability, neurological impairment, perceptual impairment, hyperactivity, and attention-deficit disorder. Unfortunately, these terms are loosely and variously defined with the result that significant confusion exists regarding a wide range of issues relevant to them. However, most agree that the entities that we are dealing with here have a greater neurological loading than psychogenic disorders—which are generally considered to be primarily, if not exclusively, induced by psychological factors in the environment.

In this volume I first present the definitions of the aforementioned terms that appear most reasonable to me. I then describe in detail a theory of the causes of these disorders. The theory is a comprehensive one, which I considered applicable to more than 95% of children who exhibit these symptoms. The theory also describes the relationships between these seemingly disparate symptoms.

In the second part of the book I describe a study that was originally designed to find a pencil-and-paper test that could be useful for assessing objectively the effects of psycho-stimulant medication. The purpose was to find an instrument that could be used by the clinician, in an office or clinical setting, to monitor psychostimulant medication. I considered the need for such an instrument to be great, because of the many problems attendant to the common practice of diagnosing hyperactivity and attention-deficit disorder (ADD) with subjective criteria only. Although I was unsuccessful in finding such an instrument, the results of the study proved to be useful in providing confirmation of some of the aspects of the theory presented in the earlier part of the book. Thus the placement of all the material in the same volume.

I consider the theory presented here to provide a meaningful explanation for what appears to be a wide variety of disparate phenomena. I believe also that it has important implications for our understanding of hyperactivity and ADD—both of which are overdiagnosed and one of which (ADD) probably doesn't exist. My hope is that the reader who has responded with surprise and even incredulity to my statement about the non-existence of ADD will at least have second thoughts about the concept after reading this book. Ideally, I would hope that such a reader will be brought to the point of agreement with me that the term should be dispensed with entirely because it describes a non-phenomenon.

ONE

The Basic Theory of the Etiology of the Group of Minimal Brain Dysfunction Syndromes

INTRODUCTION

I present here a theory of the etiology of minimal brain dysfunction. Actually, I prefer to use the term *The Group of Minimal Brain Dysfunction Syndromes* (GMBDS) because we are not dealing with a single disease entity; rather, we are dealing with a group of syndromes. A syndrome, by definition, is a cluster of symptoms that warrant being grouped together as an entity because of one or more common etiological factors. Accordingly, there are certain symptom clusters that can appear as manifestations of a variety of diseases. And when we are talking about minimal brain dysfunction, we do well to consider there to be a group of syndromes, each of which may be a manifestation of a variety of disease entities. There is good reason to believe that with advances in medical science we will come to learn more about the wide variety of specific disease entities that are incorporated under the GMBDS rubric.

This seemingly complex concept may not be as mind-boggling as it may initially appear in that the vast majority of children who exhibit GMBDS manifestations fall into only one etiological category which, I suspect, includes over 95% of the children so diagnosed. The remaining etiological factors (and they are multiple and many of them are still unknown) comprise approximately 5%. These figures are not based on any statistical studies; rather they are based on approximately 30 years' experience observing and studying these children. The theory I present here to explain the cause in this 95% group is very much my own. Although I would suspect that others have derived the same concept from their own experiences, I have not yet seen it published, nor have I heard the concept spoken about. I consider the theory to be a reasonable one—a theory which, I believe, pulls together a wide variety of seemingly disparate phenomena. My hope is that it will seem reasonable to the reader as well.

FIVE AREAS OF NEUROLOGICAL FUNCTIONING IN WHICH THE HUMAN BEING FAR SURPASSES THE HIGHER APE

Logical Reasoning

For the purposes of this presentation I will focus on 5 areas of neurological functioning in which the human being differs significantly from higher apes. The first is *logical reasoning*. Although one might train a higher ape to solve the simplest logical problems, it is not likely that even the "genius" ape will surpass the reasoning capacity of the average 2- to 3-year-old—even after years of arduous laboratory training. The human being's capacity for conceptualization and abstract thinking far surpasses that of any lower animal and is responsible for some of the marvels of our modern technological society. (I am not addressing myself to the *value* of these technological phenomena, only to the fact that ingenious cognitive processes were necessary for their development.) It is probable that the frontal lobes, more than any other part of the brain, are the sites of such cognitive processes and this is related to the fact that our frontal lobes are so much more highly developed than those of the higher apes and all other lower animals.

Visual Processing

The second area of neurological functioning in which the human being surpasses all other forms of life is in the capacity to *process visual information*. Our eyes are very similar neuroanatomically to those of the higher apes and even the tracts that extend from the retina to the occipital cortex are almost identical. However, when one then follows visual impulses anteriorly, into the complex association tracts and the various connections between visual systems and those of other brain functions, it is clear that the human brain is far more complex than that of lower animals and capable of many more sophisticated functions.

Probably the most obvious manifestation of this superiority in visual processing is the human being's capacity to read written language. By *language* I refer to the capacity to form a link between an entity and a written symbol which is used to denote specifically that entity. There is generally no intrinisic relationship between the entity and the written symbol, but social convention defines such linkage. For example, there is no intrinsic relationship between the object that we refer to in the English language as a glass and the written word *glass*. When the first-grade teacher writes the word *glass* under the picture of this object she hopes that the children will link the written symbol with the object that it denotes. If she is successful, the picture can subsequently be removed and when the word *glass* is displayed a visual image of the object will appear in the child's mind. This is the central element in the phenomenon we call *reading*. Without the ability to form an internal mental display that is linked accurately to the associated visual symbol (the written word), the individual cannot be said to be able to read. One might be able to teach a higher ape to recognize a few simple words, but a bright 3-year-old can be taught this capacity in a relatively short period and will exhibit a facility with this function that could never be achieved by an ape—even after years of intensive training. Language, although the most complex, is only one of a variety of visual processing functions. In Chapter Two I will discuss some of these other visual functions, both with regard to similarities' and differences between the human being and the higher ape. Such comparisons are important if one is to appreciate the nature of the deficiencies suffered by GMBDS children.

Auditory Processing

The third area of neurological functioning in which the human being surpasses the higher ape is that of *auditory processing*. Our ears are anatomically very similar to those of many other lower forms of life and the pathways that lead from the internal ear to the temporal lobes are also almost identical in all higher (and even many lower) forms of life. Again, it is what happens to the auditory impulses after they reach the temporal cortex that differentiates the human being from even the most sophisticated higher animals. This difference is best demonstrated by comparing the human being's capacity for auditory linguistic functioning with that of the higher ape.

By *auditory language* I refer to the capacity to form a linkage between an entity and the acoustical symbol that by social definition has been devised to denote that entity. Returning to the example of the glass, there is no intrinsic relationship between the physical entity glass and the sounds of the spoken word *glass*. Yet, if one is to understand what another person is saying, one has to be able to appreciate this socially devised linkage. When mother gives her 2-year-old boy a glass of milk and tells him that he is now old enough to drink his milk from a glass, she is teaching the child to form a link between the object she is holding in her hand and the word *glass* that she is speaking. A first-grade teacher draws a picture of a glass on the blackboard and writes the word *glass* underneath it. She simultaneously says to the children: "This is the way you spell *glass*." Her hope here is that the child will appreciate a triangular kind of linkage, that is, between the written word *glass*, the spoken word *glass*, and the entity which both the visual and the auditory symbols denote. Accordingly, when the picture is removed, *seeing* the written symbol should elicit the visual-mental display and *hearing* the auditory symbol should elicit the same visual-mental entity. Furthermore, hearing the acoustical symbol should enable the child to write the visual equivalent, that is, *write* the word (hopefully correctly spelled).

The ability to appreciate these complex relationships among an entity and its complex visual and auditory linguistic equivalents enable the human being to perform functions that are far more sophisticated than higher apes can possibly accomplish. Understanding spoken language, although the most complex form of auditory functioning, is only one of a wide variety of auditory processing functions. I will discuss in Chapter Two some of the other types of auditory processing, with particular focus on the differences between the human being and other animals. Again, it is through an understanding of these differences that one is in a better position to understand the kinds of deficits exhibited by GMBDS children.

Speech

The fourth area of neurological functioning in which the human being surpasses significantly all other forms of life is that of *speech*. It is important to differentiate *speech* from *language*.

Speech refers to the capacity to articulate language. The two functions are obviously intimately related but they are also quite separate. Language is primarily a cerebral function whereas speech, although it has its origins in the brain, is primarily a peripheral neuromuscular function in which the mouth, pharynx, and larynx are primarily involved. Years of training might enable a higher ape to utter a few distinguishable sounds. But the human being's capacity for forming a wide variety of sophisticated and recognizably different sounds is immense. There are individuals who can speak 30 or more languages. When one compares the speech area in the posterior inferior frontal lobe of the human brain with that of the higher ape the differences regarding size and neuroanatomic complexity are impressive.

Fine Motor Coordination

The fifth area of neurological functioning in which the human being differs significantly from lower animals is in the realm of *fine motor coordination*. The higher ape cannot oppose serially the tip of the thumb to the tips of each of the other 4 fingers, nor can the newborn infant. The capacity to do this develops within the first few years of life. Although this may not appear initially to be an important difference, it is actually a formidable one. If not for this capacity we humans could not write, play a wide variety of musical instruments, paint masterpieces, build sophisticated machinery, fly airplanes, maneuver space ships, and perform the wide variety of other complex functions that are responsible for a civilized technological society. We could still, however, wield clubs and throw rocks, just like the higher apes and the earliest forms of human being. The anterior portion of the parietal lobe, where such functions are represented in the brain, is significantly more developed in the human being than in the higher ape.

THE THREE BELL-SHAPED CURVES

The Adult Distribution Curve

It is reasonable to assume that for each of the wide variety of functions subsumed under each of the aforementioned 5 categories there exists a bell-shaped curve with regard to an individual's facility. For example, with regard to auditory differentiation (one of the auditory processing functions), there are some individuals who have perfect pitch and are able to recognize and identify any note on the piano; there are others who are "tone deaf" and could not do this even after a lifetime of training. And the vast majority of individuals fall at some point between these two extremes. Some can learn 35 languages and others have formidable difficulty learning even a few hundred words in their native tongue. Most fall somewhere between these extremes. In the realm of fine motor coordination, there are some who can learn to type with amazing speed and others who will never be able to develop more than the most rudimentary capacity with the typewriter. The distributions referred to here are those for adults and relate to the wide range of functioning that extends from the weakest to the strongest, with the largest number of individuals lying somewhere between the two extremes. This distribution refers to the first of the three bell-shaped curves that one must consider in understanding the deficits of GMBDS children. I refer to this first bell-shaped curve as *the adult distribution curve*.

The Individual's Personal Series of Developmental Curves

The second series of bell-shaped curves relates to each individual's areas of neurological development. I believe that the age at which an individual will exhibit a specific capacity is primarily determined by genetic factors. Some individuals will exhibit a particular capacity at a younger age and others at a relatively older age. Some children will walk without support at 9 months, others not until 16 months, but the majority do so at 12-14 months. All, however, may be in the normal range. Some children can tie their shoelaces at age 2 and others cannot perform this function until age 11 or 12. And the same principle applies for the ability to appreciate the linkages necessary to understand meaningful linguistic communication. One child can learn to read at age 2 and another not until 10. Both, however, may ultimately read with the same degree of sophistication and understanding. The former may be called "a genius" at age 2 and the latter "a dyslexic" at age 9. If one were to chart the number of children who perform each of these functions at the ages at which they exhibited the capacity, one would also obtain a bell-shaped curve. Every individual's personal developmental milestones fall on points on each of a vast number of bell-shaped curves. Children with GMBDS are likely to fall between 1 and 2 standard deviations below the mean on many of these curves, especially the curves related to the aforementioned 5 areas of of neurological functioning. I refer to these curves as *the individual's personal series of developmental curves.*

The Curves of Evolutionary Progression

The Shift to the Right of the Curves of Evolutionary Progression   Another factor to be considered is that of evolution. Mention has been made of the primitive human being's ability to throw rocks and wield clubs and inability to perfom sophisticated fine motor functions. Obviously, the latter capacity developed over time and at each point in evolution there was a bell-shaped curve among individuals reflecting the capacities of human beings with regard to fine motor functions. One could speculate that there was a time that the average individual who could justifiably be called "a human being" had the capacity to understand 100 words with the range extending from a few words to a few hundred words. Over the past hundreds of thousands of years humans expanded their capacities with regard to this function so that there was probably another time when the average person could understand 500 words with the range going from a few words to a few thousand. And, at the present time the average person on earth probably understands a few thousand words with the range extending from a few words to a few hundred thousand. Accordingly, one could envision over the course of evolution a *shift to the right of the mean* of any distribution curve for any particular function. It is reasonable to assume that an important factor in such a shift was the process of natural selection by which there was a selective survival of those who were more facile with a particular function. I refer to this phenomenon as the *shift to the right of the curves of evolutionary progression*.

The Narrowing and Stabilization of the Curves of Evolutionary Progression   It is reasonable to speculate that an important determinant of where on a particular bell-shaped curve an individual's functioning capacity will lay relates to the errors in development that must inevitably take place with complex functions. It is obvious that the more complex a neurological system, the greater the number of nerve cells necessary to perform the function, and the greater the likelihood of error at every level of development. When there are only a few thousand nerve cells involved in performing a simple function (the case for lower animals) there is far less likelihood of developmental error than for a function which may involve billions of nerve cells (the case for humans).

This principle is well demonstrated by comments I read many years ago in a pamphlet of advice on the purchase of a washing machine. Basically, the author pointed out to the would-be purchaser that the the greater the number of functions the washing machine is able to perform, the greater the number of dials and buttons there will be, the more expensive will be the machine, and the greater the number of trips by the repairman. In contrast, the fewer the number of possible functions the machine can perform, the fewer will be the number of buttons and dials, the less will be the cost, and the fewer will be the expected trips by the repairman. This obvious principle is applicable to the human brain as well regarding the risks that are entailed in the evolutionary progression to increased complexity. It is reasonable to speculate, as well, that when a more complex function first appears, many variations arise, some of which are quite useful and others less so—but may still survive (although less preferentially). These factors probably result in a low flat distribution curve for the more recently developed and sophisticated functions—a curve that reflects the wide range of capacities among individuals. With the passage of time, individuals carrying genes for the maladaptive extremes, that is, those individuals who possess variations that are less adaptable to a particular environment do not survive. This results in a narrowing of the bell-shaped curve with regard to that particular function. Accordingly, functions which we share in common with lower animals, such as pain, temperature, light touch and other spinal cord functions are probably represented by a high narrow bell-shaped curve because the extremes have not been permitted to selectively survive. The same process has been accompanied by a stabilizing of the function as it becomes increasingly efficient with regard to its being programmed into the genetic structure. Children with GMBDS generally do not have problems that are manifestations of primitive spinal cord dysfunction. (GMBDS children are to be distinguished from cerebral palsied children who often do exhibit spinal cord dysfunction, but CP children have more massive brain dysfunction than those with GMBDS.) GMBDS children, however, do have difficulties with the more recently developed, more complex functions because 1) with greater neurological complexity there is a greater likelihood of developmental error and 2) these recently developed systems have not gone through the process of selective survival and entrenchment into the neurological structure. I refer to this phenomenon as *the narrowing and stabilization of the curves of evolutionary progression.*

It may be that in the 20th century, for the first time, we are altering the natural evolutionary process with regard to the functions being discussed here. We are allowing the survival of individuals who probably did not survive in earlier times. In the more competitive "dog-eat-dog" world that existed up to the present, the kinds of people who exhibited what I have referred to as GMBDS were not given the kind of protection, guidance, sympathetic understanding, and education that we are providing such individuals today. This was especially the case in large industrial complexes where such individuals were certainly less capable of surviving in the more sophisticated and competitive environment; it was less the case in the agrarian environment. Accordingly, GMBDS individuals are more likely to survive now and procreate— and transmit thereby their deficits. I am not suggesting that we do otherwise; I am only stating what I consider to be the result of our humanitarian efforts, namely, that we are reversing the evolutionary narrowing of the bell-shaped distribution curve. The phenomenon is not new to medicine. All attempts to enable children with genetically based diseases to survive to the age when they can procreate results in an increase of disease-producing genes in the genetic pool.

Final Comments on the Three Bell-Shaped Curves

In short, then, when considering the important genetic factors operative in the development of the GMBDS, one must consider simultaneously a number of bell-shaped curves. One must take into consideration the distribution of the particular function among adults (the adult distribution curve), and recognize that among adults there is a wide variety of functioning capacity—from the weakest to the strongest. One must take into consideration each individual's own personal development and recognize that there is a wide variety of ages at which children will exhibit facility with a particular function (the individual's personal series of developmental curves). In addition, one must recognize that many late developers will be no different from early developers by the time they reach adulthood. One must consider, as well, the fact that the mean capacity of all individuals at any particular time for any particular function is shifting to the right over the passage of time (the curves of evolutionary progression). Another way of viewing these evolutionary factors is to consider some individuals as being 100,000 years or so behind others. For example, an individual with a linguistic capacity of 500 words is certainly significantly below average in the 20th century, was average at some point in the past, and was above average at some remote time in the distant past. Last, the process of narrowing and stabilization of the evolutionary distribution curves must be considered in that the child with GMBDS may be viewed as possessing genes that might not have been permitted survival in more viciously competitive and inhumane times.

Many readers, I am sure, are familiar with the famous lines from Shakespeare's *As You Like It*:

> All the world's a stage,
> And all the men and women merely players:
> They have their exits and their entrances;
> And each man, in his time, plays many parts . . . .

With all due respect to Mr. William Shakespeare, I believe that his concept is a narrow one. I myself view it this way:

> All the world's a bell-shaped curve,
> And all the men and women merely numbers:
> They have their means and their standard deviations;
> And each man, in his time, appears on many curves.

THE RELATIONSHIPS BETWEEN THE AFOREMENTIONED BELL-SHAPED CURVES AND THE ETIOLOGY OF THE GMBDS

I believe that these concepts serve well as an explanation for the deficits we are observing in the vast majority of children who are diagnosed as having a neurologically based learning disability. The typical child who is so diagnosed is one whose IQ is in the 85 to 95 range. The child generally has trouble learning because of auditory processing deficits, and/or visual processing deficits, and/or impairments in reasoning. Furthermore, there are often associated speech impairments as well as fine motor coordination deficiencies. For the vast majority of these children the etiology of their dificits is unknown. Although the examiner may find in the history such suspected etiological factors as prolonged labor, low birth weight, and maternal bleeding during pregnancy, there are many children with a similar history who exhibit no symptomatology in the GMBDS realm. In most cases the etiology it only surmised and the sophisticated examiner will often have some doubts as to whether there is a direct relationship between the presumed etiological factor(s) and the child's symptomatology.

I believe that the vast majority of these children have nothing more wrong with them than the fact that they are at about the 10th to 25th percentile levels on cognitive bell-shaped curves such as those to be found in the *Wechsler Intelligence Scale for Children — Revised* (WISC-R) (D. Wechsler, 1974). It is obvious that for every child with a 115 IQ there must be a child with an 85 IQ. For every child with a 110 IQ there must be a child with a 90 IQ. And it is equally clear that for every child with a 140 IQ there must be a child with a 60 IQ. Accordingly, Wechsler must have been assessing GMBDS children when the instrument was standardized. Wechsler's manual describes in detail the population used for the test's standardization and clearly states (page 19) that "Suspected mental defectives, however, were not excluded if they lived at home." What we are doing then is artificially selecting a particular segment (approximately the 10th-25th percentile) on the *normal curve* and claiming that these children are suffering with a disease. Many of these children, had they been born into an agrarian society, would not have been so designated. GMBDS children have had the misfortune of having been born in the late 20th century into a technological society where they are being pressured into succeeding in exactly those areas in which they are weakest. They have been born into a society where the educational system focuses heavily on reasoning capacity and auditory and visual processing abilities—the exact areas in which they are least likely to succeed. Moveover, they are usually required to attend school to the mid-teens, forcing them thereby to expose themselves to an environment that cannot but be psychologically detrimental—the potential benefits of their education notwithstanding. To me, it is more reasonable to say that these children have had bad luck, rather than that they suffer with a disease.

THE SO-CALLED "INTELLIGENCE TEST," ESPECIALLY AS IT RELATES TO THE DIAGNOSIS OF CHILDREN WITH GMBDS

At this point, I will make a few comments on the so-called intelligence tests. An understanding of their development will place the reader in a better position to appreciate my views on this subject, especially as they relate to understanding the problems of GMBDS children. In the early part of this century the taxpayers of Paris complained that money was being wasted on attempts to educate retarded children (then unashamedly referred to a morons, imbeciles, and idiots) in the regular classroom structure. They asked the well-known psycholgist Alfred Binet to devise a test that would help educators detect such children so that they might be removed from the regular classroom and thereby save the taxpayers money. Accordingly, Binet went into the classrooms and observed carefully what the teachers were teaching. He then developed a test based on what was bring taught in the Parisian educational system at that time. It was subsequently found that those children who did poorly on Binet's test were likely to do poorly in school and those who did well on it were likely to do well in school. Binet's test was not called an intelligence test. Rather, it was merely a test designed to predict success and failure in the educational system from which its questions were derived.In 1916 Terman, at Stanford University in California, translated the Binet test into English and revised the questions to make the test more compatible with the material being taught in American schools at that time. It was around that time that the word "intelligence" crept into the name, thus, the *Stanford-Binet Test of Intelligence* (L.M. Terman and M.A. Merrill 1937, 1960). Wechsler too used the term *intelligence* in his tests both in the original edition (1949) and the revised edition (1974). I think it would be more honest to say that these are not tests of intelligence, but tests that predict success in the school system from which the test questions were derived in the first place.

Some examples of children in other cultures will be used to demonstrate my point here. Let us imagine a child born today into a South American Indian tribe, completely remote from industrialized society. In order to succeed in such a tribe, the child has to be able to differentiate visually between the footprints of various animals. This not only serves well hunting purposes but may have survival value in that it enables the youngster to differentiate between friendly animals and those that may be predatory. The youngster must be able to differentiate well between the sounds of different animals, again for the purpose of distinguishing between friendly and hostile species. Olfactory sensitivity is also important. The odors of animals, their droppings, and lingering smells are important to differentiate in such an environment. The development of various physical skills is also important: building fires, constructing shelters, utilizing weapons and hunting instruments, and knowing how to fight. Clearly, if one were going to devise a "test of intelligence" for youngsters in this tribe one would want to base it on things being taught in "Indian School." The more honest name for the test would be: a test to predict success in the Indian educational system from which the test questions were derived. It is conceivable that children whose genetic programming would enable them to succeed well in an industrialized society's schools would not have done well in "Indian schools" and vice versa. Of course, there are children whose genetic programming is such that they would do well in both school systems and others who would do poorly in both educational programs.

Now to another example. Let us envision a child born today into an agrarian society in a subculture of farm laborers. From birth the child and his or her family knows that only simple farm tasks will be required. (I am not addressing myself here to whether absence of potential for "upward mobility" in this society is good or bad, only its relevance to the understanding of GMBDS). In order to "succeed" in this society the child only needs to learn how to do such things as pick fruits off a tree, do simple plowing, pull vegetables out of the earth, and perform other simple tasks. Although the child's genetic programming may be such that, if born into a Western industrialized society, he or she might have been a mathematics professor, such potential skills are not being utilized and thereby brought into maximum expression. But, if in that society, a child's genetic programming is such that he or she would be designated as having GMBDS in our society, the child will suffer no discomfort because the agrarian environment is not making demands on those areas that are weak. Such a child will function well in an agrarain society and not suffer the ego-debasing experiences that GMBDS children suffer in ours. My main point here is that for the majority of children with GMBDS the view that they have a disease—with the implication that there is something intrinsically pathological in their central nervous systems—is an artifact of our highly industrialized society and is thereby a terrible disservice to these children.

GMBDS CHILDREN IN WHOM BRAIN NEUROPATHOLOGY IS ACTUALLY PRESENT

Now to carry this theory a bit furthur, to include the aforementioned remaining 5% or so who are diagnosed GMBDS. I believe that in this small group are children who actually did sustain some medical trauma that did indeed bring about neurological damage. This damage sits on top of the aforementioned genetically determined neurological substrata. In some of these children their genetic programming dictated that they be at the lower end of certain bell-shaped curves that are under consideration in making the GMBDS diagnosis. Others were programmed to be in the middle of many such curves and still others at the upper ends. However, the superimposed disease process has depressed neurological functioning, with the result that their potentials have been lowered. These are children for whom the etiology is considered to be known. In pregnancy, some of the factors that are generally considered to be of etiological significance are infection, especially toxoplasmosis, rubella, syphilis, and cytomegalic virus infection (which may be asymptomatic in the mother and not manifest itself in the child until he or she attends school). Toxemia of pregnancy has also been implicated.

Smoking during pregnancy has been associated with low birth weight, increased fetal and neonatal death rate, and impairments in the child's physical, neurological, and intellectual growth. And there appears to be a correlation between the amount of smoking and the incidence of these effects. Excessive alcoholic ingestion can cause what has been referred to as the *fetal alcohol syndrome*. These babies exhibit alterations in growth, facial dysmorphism and other disturbances of body morphogenesis, as well as low birth weight. GMBDS and mental retardation have been described in these children. Drugs ingested by the mother that have been known to cause brain dysfunction in the child include aminopterin, phenytoin, methotrexate, cocaine (and other narcotics), and high doses of vitamin D. And there are probably many other drugs, as yet unimplicated, that will ultimately be shown to have such effects. A standard warning provided for a high percentage of drugs is that safe administration during pregnancy has not been established. Accordingly, any medication that was taken over a period during the pregnancy should be noted by the examiner. Exposure to X-radiation has also been implicated. A woman presents with symptoms of nausea, vomiting, and other gastrointestinal symptoms. Pregnancy may not be suspected, especially if the woman is single or over 40. The patient may have undergone a number of radiological examinations (GI series, gall bladder studies, barium enema, etc.) in the attempt to ascertain the cause of the vomiting. By the time the correct diagnosis is made, the woman may have been exposed to significant amounts of X-radiation. (Most radiologists now inquire into the recent menstrual history to be sure that they are not exposing a pregnant woman to X-rays.)

There are a variety of genetic and/or congenital neurological disorders that have been associated with brain dysfunction. Probably the most common of these is Down's syndrome. Furthermore, brain dysfunction is also likely to be associated with those disorders that directly involve the central nervous system and/or the tissues and bones in which it is encased. The most common disorders in this category are meningocele, meningomyelocele, meningoencephalocele, hydrocephalus, and spina bifida. Fortunately, techniques have been developed in recent years for detecting the presence of the aforementioned disorders during the course of the pregnancy. The most recently developed technique in this realm is *chorionic villi sampling* (CVS). This is generally done during the first trimester, usually in the 8th to 10th week of pregnancy. Chorionic material is snipped and aspirated via the cervical approach. Because the chorionic villi are essentially fetal cells, they can allow for a complete chromosome analysis of the fetus. Accordingly, Down's syndrome and other chromosomal abnormalities can be detected at this early stage of the pregnancy. In addition, the aspirate can be analyzed for alpha-fetal proteins that are likely to be present in very high concentrations when an *open* neural tube defect is present— such as in some of the aforementioned neurological cranial and spinal cord disorders.

During the 16th to 18th week of pregnancy one can utilize amniocentesis to obtain the same information. Here, the aspirate examined is that of the amniotic fluid that is obtained by direct aspiration through the abdominal and uterine walls. It is during this period that the mother's serum may also contain high levels of alpha-fetal proteins, thereby allowing for diagnosis of fetal neural tube defects without direct examination of the fetus and its environment. A sonogram can also diagnose hydrocephalus during this period.

Chorionic villi sampling has many advantages over amniocentesis. CVS is a 1st trimester procedure and thereby provides information at a much earlier point in the pregnancy; whereas amniocentesis is a 2nd trimester procedure. If the mother elects to abort the child it can be easily accomplished in the first trimester with dilatation and curetage (D & C). In contrast, if the mother elects to abort following 2nd trimester amniocentesis studies, the procedure for inducing abortions is more complex, has a higher risk (still quite small, however), and is more psychologically stressful because of the similarity between the aborted fetus during this period and the newborn. Second trimester abortion is generally accomplished by inducing labor. This is generally done by the direct injection of saline solution or prostaglandin into the amniotic sac or the insertion of prostaglandin suppositories into the vagina. These procedures are likely to be far more psychologically traumatic to the mother than a 1st trimester D & C.

The time of delivery is another period when the child may be exposed to factors that can produce GMBDS. Inducing labor runs certain risks for the child, more so in the past than in the present. The physician may miscalculate the pregnancy's duration (especially if he or she relies too heavily on the mother's estimate) and deliver the baby before it can thrive optimally in the extrauterine environment. In the past oxytocin, the drug most commonly used to initate and maintain uterine contractions, was administered by buccal tablet. One had no control over the duration of its action. Accordingly, uterine contractions might persist after it was determined that cephalopelvic disproportion was present and the fetus was being traumatized. In addition, drugs such as oxytocin can produce tetanic contractions of the uterus. These can cut off blood circulation from the placenta to the fetus and thereby cause anoxia in the child. Since the early 1970s oxytocin is given only by intravenous drip, which can be carefully controlled. Once trouble is suspected, the oxytocin is immediately discontinued. Because there is no reserve of the drug present in the body (as is the case with buccal tablets) uterine contractions due to the drug can be quickly interrupted. The mother who is spontaneously delivered does not run the risk of these complications.

The onset of labor contractions may cause or precipitate various forms of fetal distress—distress that may be associated with a variety of disorders which can affect brain functioning. Some of the more common are head trauma, compression of the umbilical cord, toxemia, and other disorders related to maternal high blood pressure and/or an aged placenta. One of the most sensitive manifestations of fetal distress is a deceleration of the fetal heart rate. Accordingly, obstetricians traditionally listen to the fetal heart with their stethoscopes during the course of the labor in order to ascertain whether fetal distress is present. Unfortunately, this traditional technique is compromised significantly by the fact that the fetal heart rate is generally not audible during uterine contractions. Accordingly, the event (uterine contractions) that is most likely to result in decelerization of the fetal heart rate interferes with the procedure (auscultation of the fetal heart) that is designed to detect such deceleration. Furthermore, it is unreasonable to expect the obstetrician and/or other personnel attending to a woman in labor to constantly attempt to monitor the fetal heart rate. Rather, such examinations are usually intermittent and often miss those times when the heart rate temporarily decelerates. Accordingly, the emergency cesarean deliveries that were often indicated upon the presence of such signs of fetal distress were not performed and babies were born with a variety of complications, one of which was brain damage.

Fortunately, more recent advances have improved significantly the efficacy of monitoring for fetal distress. Specifically, a variety of electronic instruments have been devised which *constantly* provide monitoring, thereby alerting those in attendance to any transient deceleration of the fetal heart. In addition, maternal and fetal events are monitored *separately*, obviating thereby the aforementioned interference with hearing the fetal heart by the contracting uterus. The mother's contractions are monitored externally by a pressure gauge placed on the abdomen at the fundus of the uterus. The fetus' heart can be monitored externally by the utilization of a Sonar-Doplar technique. It can be monitored internally by the placement of an electrode on the emerging baby's scalp. These new monitoring techniques have enabled obstetrician's to interrupt fetal distress, generally by performing a cesarean section, and thereby lessen the likelihood that the fetus will suffer from the causes of the distress. Whereas head trauma incurred during labor was a common cause of brain damage in the past, it no longer is so because of fetal monitoring and cesarean section, when indicated.

Breech deliveries are generally more traumatic than vertex. Cesarean sections, especially those that are resorted to because of complications that have interfered with delivery via the birth canal, have also been associated with GMBDS. It is probable that it was not the cesarean section *per se* that caused the GMBDS, but the complications that caused the obstetrician to utilize this method of delivery. When a child is born with a "nuchal cord," i.e. with the umbilical cord twisted around the neck, there may have been some compromise of blood circulation from the placenta to the fetal brain. However, only a small percentage of infants who present with a nuchal cord have been found to be brain damaged; most suffer no sequelae from this potential complication. When the cord presents first, there may be compression of the blood circulation to the infant, because the baby's head compresses the umbilical cord as it moves down the birth canal. This results in impairment of circulation to the infant's brain. Excessive blood loss during labor may also reduce the amount of blood reaching the infant.

Birth weight is no longer considered to be the criterion of prematurity. In fact, most neonatologists discourage the use of the term prematurity. Low-birth-weight babies, that is, those weighing less than 2500 grams, are divided into two categories: 1) those whose birth weights are appropriate for their gestational age (AGA) and 2) those whose weights are low, that is, they are small for gestational age (SGA). We now have objective physiological and neurological criteria for determining gestational age and do not have to rely on a mother's recollection of when she thinks she became pregnant. The babies in these 2 groups are quite different. Consider, for example, two babies whose birth weight is 1500 grams. One baby is found to have a gestational age of 31 weeks and the other 37 weeks. Because 1500 grams is about normal for 31 week fetuses, the first baby would be considered AGA. The second would be considered SGA. The assumption is made that the second baby has only grown to the 31 week size in a 37 week pregnancy. Something has happened to retard the child's growth. The second child is more likely to exhibit difficulties that would include GMBDS. The first is more likely to develop normally in that nothing serious is considered to have happened to it, although its low birth weight is still an abnormality that may cause difficulty.

Babies of large size (over 9 pounds) are also at greater risk for the development of GMBDS, in that their deliveries are more likely to be traumatic. Babies of long gestation (over 42 weeks) are also likely to have complications such as GMBDS because the aging placenta becomes more inefficient in its functioning and meconium aspiration is also more likely in such infants. The malfunctioning placenta causes distress in the fetus. One manifestation of such fetal distress is relaxation of the anal sphincter which, in turn, produces passage of meconium into the amniotic sac. This in turn becomes aspirated and results in fetal asphyxia.

The healthy child breathes spontaneously at birth. At most, the child requires some clearing of the nasal passages. The traditional slap to get the child breathing is considered by most obstetricians to be unnecessary. The usual nasopharyngeal aspiration provides enough stimulation to induce breathing. The longer the delay in breathing the greater the likelihood the child will suffer with cerebral anoxemia. The normal infant spontaneously cries at birth. A delayed cry is also an index of infant depression, especially of respiration and bodily response to stimulation. A fairly objective statement about the newborn's overall physical condition at the time of birth is the Apgar score (V. Apgar, 1953; V. Apgar et al., 1958). At one, two, and five minutes after birth, the child is given a score of 0, 1, or 2 on five items. The five physiological functions evaluated are heart rate, respiratory effort, muscle tone, reflex irritability, and general color. With a maximum score of 10, 2 is considered severe depression; 4, 5, 6, or 7 is moderate depression; and 8, 9, or 10 is no depression.

About 40% of newborns exhibit a transient physiologic jaundice (icterus neonatorum). There are two causes of this type of jaundice: 1) There is the increased destruction of red blood cells in order to reduce the high fetal red cell concentration (necessary for intrauterine existence) to the lower levels necessary after birth. 2) The immature liver is inefficient in its capacity to metabolize bilirubin and other products of red blood cell destruction. Generally, the jaundice appears on the 2nd to 4th day and ends between the 7th and 14th. Jaundice due to Rh incompatibility (erythroblastosis fetalis) or ABO incompatibility (icterus neonatorum) usually begins during the first 24 hours and is severer. Immunological treatment with RhoGAM (an anti-Rh + antibody globulin) can prevent Rh incompatibility disorder in mothers who have not yet been sensitized. The injection is given right after the delivery and prevents the Rh − mother from developing antibodies to her own baby's Rh + blood cells − protecting thereby subsequent Rh + babies from developing erythroblastosis fetalis. In recent years phototherapy has been found useful in the treatment of physiological jaundice as well as the milder forms of jaundice due to ABO incompatibility. And RhoGAM has been successful in preventing entirely the severer forms of jaundice related to Rh incompatibility. Children whose mothers may not have received these treatments may develop brain damage as a result of their hyperbilirubinemia. The most common kind of brain damage caused by high bilirubin levels is the kernicterus resulting from icteric degeneration of the basal ganglia as well as other cerebral centers.

Cyanosis is a concomitant of anoxia, which may cause nerve cell dysfunction and degeneration. Anoxia may be seen in prematurity in association with the respiratory distress syndrome (hyaline membrane disease), maternal toxemia, and any other condition in which the neonate is under stress. Cyanosis may also result from intracranial hemorrhage, which is sometimes caused by birth trauma or hemmorrhagic disease of the newborn. In some cases the etiology of the intracranial bleeding is unknown. Congenital atalectasis, hyaline membrane disease, and various congenital heart diseases can also cause cyanosis. The need for incubator care may be a clue to the presence of apnea, cyanosis, and a variety of diseases affecting respiration and circulation.

Congenital cardiac anomalies may also be associated with cerebral nerve cell degeneration. This is especially true of the cyanotic forms that are associated with hypoxic spells such as the tetralogy of Fallot. The noncyanotic forms are not directly associated with brain dysfunction, but could be indirectly associated because of the presence of arrhythmias, coma, and heart failure.

One must consider the wide variety of childhood diseases that can bring about cerebral impairment. Traditional childhood diseases, such as measles and mumps, were on rare occasion associated with central nervous system complications such as encephalitis. Fortunately, with the advent of new vaccines, we are seeing much less of these disorders. A history of coma and/or seizures associated with such an illness is suggestive of central nervous system involvement even though medical attention may not have been sought.

Investigation into past surgical procedures may provide a clue to the etiology. For example, the child with frequent bouts of otitis media requiring myringotomies is suspect for hearing impairment which may interfere with speech and learning. There is hardly a child who does not sustain occasional head trauma. But when it is associated with unconsciousness or coma, then brain dysfunction (not necessarily permanent) must be suspected.

There was a time when a child who only had seizures with fever was considered to be neurologically normal. The child was considered to have "febrile seizures," which were not taken as seriously as those that occurred in the afebrile state. One reflection of this relaxed attitude toward febrile convulsions was the view that such seizures did not warrant anticonvulsant medication. The traditional treatment of such seizures was to warn the parent to give the child elixir phenobarbital (or other anticonvulsant medication) as soon as the child showed signs of illness—especially a febrile illness. Unfortunately, children have a way of spiking fevers so rapidly that parents were often unaware that the child was getting sick and so did not often give the anticonvulsant in time to prevent the convulsion. Some pediatric neurologists today take such seizures more seriously. They hold that in addition to the basic pathology that causes the seizures, a seizure *per se* can result in superimposed damage to the brain. A grand mal seizure includes an apneic phase and this can cause cerebral hypoxia. Accordingly, a child with febrile seizures may be placed on maintenance anticonvulsant medication if there is a family history of seizures, signs of organic cerebral dysfunction, or other factors indicative of a high risk of additional brain dysfunction. Other pediatric neurologists hold that there has never been convincing evidence of a relationship between untreated febrile seizures and intellectual impairment. They would only put a child on anticonvulsant medication if there were present what they considered to be high risk factors for the presence of neurological impairment, e.g. an abnormal electroencephlogram, positive neurological signs, or a strong family history of a seizure disorder.

Meningitis and encephalitis, especially when associated with coma, is highly correlated with residual brain damage and is one of the more generally accepted causes of GMBDS. Encephalitides are also known to be a concomitant of untoward immunization reactions. There are some children who easily run persistently high fevers with practically any infection. Others may manifest such fevers without known cause. Children with fevers of unknown etiology may have some kind of neurophysiological dysfunction which is akin to and possibly a symptom of GMBDS. The same factors that have produced neurophysiological abnormalities in other parts of the brain may be causing impaired functioning of temperature regulatory mechanisms. Ear disorders, such as chronic infections, can involve the brain. The child who has trouble hearing or trouble understanding what he or she hears may not only have some disorder of the external ear but of the central auditory processing mechanisms as well.

Although lead has been implicated more than other substances as an etiological factor in GMBDS, the ingestion of other substances must be considered. The impulsivity, poor judgment, and intellectual impairment of GMBDS children makes them more likely to ingest drugs, poisons, and other dangerous substances. Accordingly, poisons should not only be viewed as primary etiological agents, but as potentially causing superimposed brain damage as well.

When investigating for the etiology of the GMBDS process, most examiners generally consider only the aforementioned external neurological traumas and not the neurologically based substrates on which the trauma is super-imposed. Many do, however, consider family history and make note of the fact that a relative had learning difficulties in school. The genetic factor therefore is considered but not to the depth and extent described here. Rather, the child's GMBDS is viewed as a pathological genetic trait passed down from or exhibited by the allegedly afflicted relative.

Both the aforementioned complex genetically deter-mined neurological substrate and the possible external brain insults (pre-, peri-, and postnatal) must be considered in un-derstanding the etiology of the child's deficits. I have seen children with extremely bright parents who have exhibited manifestations of GMBDS, yet their full scale IQs were not de-pressed below average. Some of these children had verbal IQs in the 140 range and performance IQs in the average range. My assumption here was that some superimposed trauma lowered fucntioning artificially (perhaps in the right brain) so that they were not reaching their genetically determined po-tentials. I have also seen children, both of whose parents had high IQs, whose IQs were depressed down to the normal range on both the verbal and performance scales of the WISC-R. Although one could simply speculate that these chil-dren's average IQs reflected genetic programming inherited from ancestors with average intelligence, one must also con-sider the possibility that they were genetically programmed to have higher intelligence (the more likely possibility for chil-dren born of 2 extremely bright parents) and that some external noxious influence lowered their intelligence. In some cases the noxious influence was readily identified; in other cases it could not be. The implications of this concept, then, are that children whose parents are highly intelligent are less likely to be intellectually impaired by superimposed noxious traumas than those whose parents are in the average or below average range of intelligence. My experience supports this assumption, but I would readily admit that it is only an assumption.

TWO

ELABORATION OF
THE BASIC THEORY

DEFINITION OF TERMS

One of the problems that exists in the GMBDS field is the variety of terms which are variously defined by different examiners. Such a state of affairs produces errors in communication, unnecessary confusion, and compromises significantly our understanding of the various processes that are operative. Accordingly, at this point I will define what I mean by the various terms frequently utilized. I am not claiming that the definitions I am using are what these entities really *are*. No one can say that his or her definition is the *correct one*. There are no tablets in heaven on which the correct definitions of these terms are etched. Rather, I present here what I consider to be reasonable definitions of these terms. These definitions, however, are not completely self-created; rather, they are related to some of the commonly used concepts that are prevalent. They are presented here to avoid the aforementioned confusion and will enable the reader to know exactly what I am talking about when I use each of these terms.

Before presenting my definitions, I believe it is important to apprise the reader of my views on the uses of the terms *psychogenic* and *organic*. Psychogenic psychopathology generally refers to disorders that are usually considered to be derived from psychologically unhealthy environmental exposures. The general consensus is that there is no specific organic brain pathology causing these disorders. Accordingly, microscopic and biochemical examination of the brain would not reveal any abnormalities. Organic symptoms are considered to be manifestations of physical or metabolic abnormalities in the brain. Sometimes these can readily be identified and other times they cannot. However, when the latter is true, the general consensus is that such pathology is present but not yet identifiable by present techniques. The theory is that because the symptoms are similar or even identical to the symptoms of diseases with demonstrable brain pathology that similar brain pathology exists in these "organic" disorders as well and that it is only a matter of time before the nature of the brain changes will be delineated and identified.

In recent years many have claimed that such a differentiation is absurd. They argue: "For every crooked thought, there must be a crooked molecule." They believe that even the most "psychogenic" symptom, that is, the one that can be completely explained as a result of psychological environmental influences, must still have a basic neurological substrate in order for the abnormal thoughts and feelings to manifest themselves. Accordingly, they believe the psychogenic/organic controversy is an anachronism, a residuum of a time when people were prone to make somewhat simplistic and artificial differentiations. I am in full agreement that there must be a "crooked molecule" for every "crooked thought." However, I am not in agreement that we should therefore dispense entirely with the psychogenic/organic differentiation. It is extremely important to try to determine *how* the molecule became crooked: whether by psychological environmental influences and/or biological mechanisms (genetic, congenital, toxic, metabolic, etc). Knowledge is power. The more we know about the causes of a disorder, the better will be our position to treat it. Molecules that got crooked from psychologically detrimental environmental exposures are more likely to be "straightened out" by changes in the environment; and molecules that got "crooked" from one or more of the aforementioned biological processes are more likely to be "straightened out" by direct influence on these processes.

Some claim that even this argument is specious because we have drugs today that straighten out crooked brain molecules regardless of the way in which they became crooked, either environmentally or biologically. I am dubious. Although many of the drugs that are being introduced today are capable of straightening out, to some extent, crooked molecules of both classes, they are not that efficacious that they do so with 100 percent efficacy. We must still address ourselves to the complex psychological, family, social, and cultural factors that are operative not only in bringing about psychogenic symptomatology but perpetuating it. An antidepressant, for example, may certainly alleviate depression in some patients; however, the medication is not likely to alter one iota the complex environmental factors that are often contributory to the symptom. Both must be addressed by therapists if they are to understand adequately the nature of the patient's disorder and provide proper treatment.

The Primary Neurological Manifestations

Figure 2-1 presents a composite of my concept of the *Group of Minimal Brain Dysfunction Syndromes*. Symptoms that are *organic* are to be found depicted *within* the large circle and those

Figure 2-1

THE GROUP OF MINIMAL BRAIN DYSFUNCTION SYNDROMES

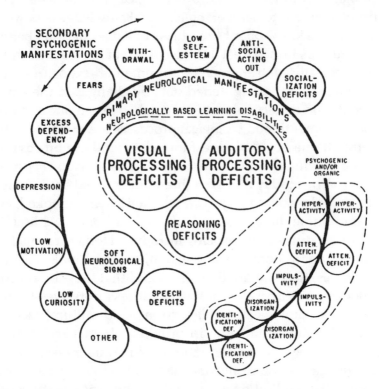

that are *psychogenic* are depicted *outside* of the largest circle. In the region of the lower right segment of the largest circle are to be found symptoms that I view to be organic and/or psychogenic and so they are portrayed twice, once inside and once outside of the circle. The disorders within the largest circle are collectively referred to as the *primary neurological manifestations.* I use the term *primary* because they are direct manifestations of neurological impairment. The symptoms depicted outside of the largest circle are referred to as the *secondary* psychogenic symptoms because they are the psychological result or derivatives of the primary deficits. I believe that if the primary neurological deficits were not present the individual would not suffer with the secondary psychogenic symptoms. Of course, these same symptoms could be derived from other sources, but that takes us beyond the purposes of this discussion. The point here is that these symptoms are likely to result when the primary neurological manifestations are present. If, however, the psychogenic symptoms appear when there are no primary neurological manifestations, then one must look to other causes of their appearance, such as environmental influences.

Within the organic group the largest and most important are the *neurologically based learning disabilities*, which is composed of *visual processing deficits, auditory processing deficits*, and *reasoning deficits*. Also to be found among the *primary neurological manifestations* are *speech deficits* and *soft neurological signs*. These represent the symptomatic manifestations of the impairments in the five areas I have discussed previously, the areas in which human beings differ significantly from higher apes. I use the term *neurologically based learning disability* synonymously with *neurological impairment (NI)*. However, I prefer the term *neurologically based learning disability* over the term *neurological impairment* because neurological impairment may refer to any kind of neurological deficit, within or outside of the central nervous system. A person with peripheral nerve weakness resulting in foot drop is suffering with a neurological impairment. In order to confine ourselves to those kinds of neurological impairments that relate to GMBDS, I prefer *neurologically based learning disability*. I generally do not use the term *perceptual impairment (PI)* because it implies a degree of purity of dysfunction that does not generally exist. Rather, when perceptual impairments are present one generally sees other GMBDS manifestations such as reasoning deficits, eye-motor coordination deficits, fine-motor coordination impairments, etc. Furthermore, the term *perceptual* is variously defined by different examiners. Some use the term to refer to speculations regarding whether the patient is seeing correctly an external visual stimulus, e.g. whether a particular geometric figure presented to the patient is actually being projected accurately on the occipital cortex. Others use the term to refer to the ability to understand the *meaning* of a particular stimulus or symbol, e.g. whether a person understands that a red light means *stop* and a green light means *go*. It is for these reasons that I avoid the term *perceptual impairment* and define more specifically the phenomenon that I am referring to.

The Secondary Psychogenic Symptoms

The child who exhibits one or more deficits in the five aforementioned areas, and who is unfortunate enough to be born into a highly industrialized society (the advantages of such a society notwithstanding), is likely to exhibit secondary psychological difficulties. Our educational systems are designed primarily to educate individuals to function successfully in the society that creates the educational program. The emphasis during the educational process is on those areas that are most likely to prove useful and necessary in the society into which the graduates will ultimately find themselves. Children with neurologically based learning disabilities are predictably going to have significant difficulty in educational systems designed to train people for adjustment in our complex technological society. The law, however, requires these children to attend school — where their defects will inevitably be exposed to peers and teachers. Predictably, such children are going to dread attending school, which becomes associated with the most mortifying experiences the child can have. Auditory processing deficits interfere with their understanding what their teachers are saying. Visual processing deficits impair their capacity to comprehend what they are reading. And impairments in reasoning interfere with their understanding what their teachers are teaching. Such children are inevitably going to develop one or more of the secondary psychogenic manifestations depicted outside of the largest circle.

Such children are likely to withdraw from peers and exhibit various *socialization deficits* because of their impairments in understanding what other children are talking about and experiencing. They do not understand the rules of games and have trouble with the concepts of sharing and sportsmanship. Their impulsivity interferes with their waiting their turns and other cognitive deficits interfere with their ability to sympathize, empathize, and put themselves in the positions of others. Their motor coordination problems interfere with their keeping up in sports. All these and other disorders contribute to these children's *socialization deficits*.

Anger is inevitably going to be engendered by the frustration and embarrassment these children feel in the classroom situation and is likely to contribute to the development of *antisocial acting out*. Furthermore, anger is engendered by the rejections the child experiences from peers, siblings, and even parents. This anger contributes to the classroom disruption that these children so often exhibit. Some GMBDS youngsters, however, suppress their anger and this contributes to the development of *anger inhibition problems*.

Low self-esteem problems are inevitable because these children cannot but help compare themselves unfavorably to peers who are more successful academically and socially. It is reasonable to say that retarded children do not have the capacity for such comparisons and so suffer less from their impairments. These children are in between. They are smarter than the retarded but less smart than the normal and those of superior intelligence. They have, however, the ability to compare themselves to others and recognize unfavorable comparisons. And this cannot but contribute to profound feelings of low self-worth. Although their parents may try to hide their disappointment, they are rarely successful in doing so. The healthy parent wants a healthy child, a child who is both physically and mentally normal. A parent cannot but be disappointed with the child who suffers with GMBDS, especially a child whose deficits cover a wide range of areas including academic, social, and recreational. However studiously such parents try to hide their disappointments, they inevitably are revealed to the child and this cannot but contribute to the child's feelings of low self-worth. In addition, normal siblings are also likely to contribute to these children's feelings of low self-esteem. They will complain that the GMBDS does not respect their privacy, embarrasses them in front of friends, often to the point where friends of the normal sibling will refuse to visit the home if the GMBDS child is present. And such rejections cannot but contribute to profound feelings of low self-worth in the GMBDS child.

GMBDS children *withdraw* from interaction with peers in order to protect themselves from the disclosure of their deficits. And they *fear* such involvement for the same reason. And such fear may generalize to a variety of situations beyond the classroom and neighborhood. For example, they may exhibit fears of the dark, new situations, strangers, being on their own, visiting other children's homes, animals, and going away to camp. They become excessively *dependent* on parents, teachers, and other authorities because of their inability to function at age-appropriate levels in a variety of areas. Such dependency relates, in part, to the fact that they do not have the ability to function at chronological age level and so regress to earlier levels of development in which they are more likely to receive assistance from adults. Such dependency is also related to the fact that their withdrawal from the world deprives them of the opportunity to acquire skills and age-appropriate levels of competence that they are physiologically capable of achieving.

Children with GMBDS are likely to become *depressed*. The prevailing notion in psychiatry today is that depression is basically a biological manifestation and that the indicated treatment is antidepressant medication. For many psychiatrists the situation is as simple as that. Some even go so far as to say that the normal healthy person will not get depressed in response to environmental traumas; only those with a specific biological impairment are likely to become depressed and require thereby andidepressant medication. I am not in agreement with this extreme position. Although I agree that there may be some genetically determined biological *predisposition* to depression, I believe that most of the depressed patients I see are so because of environmental influences and faulty thinking. Accordingly, I still believe that the vast majority of patients are depressed because of psychogenic factors; but I will agree that in a small percentage of these a genetically based biological predisposition may be present.

The depression of GMBDS children, I believe, is more reasonably explained as environmentally induced. These children have much to be depressed about. They are forced to suffer daily humiliations and indignities because of their deficits. In school, they are continually fearful of exposure of their deficits and they suffer terrible mortifications because of them. From peers, as well, they experience mostly rejection, mockery, and humiliation. Their siblings often scorn them and even their parents are disappointed in them, if not overtly rejecting. I cannot imagine an individual not becoming depressed under these circumstances. I am not denying the possible presence of a genetically based neurophysiological component to these children's depression and I am not denying that antidepressant medication may not be useful to them. I am only claiming that the largest component of their depression is more reasonably viewed as being environmentally induced and a strict biological explanation appears far less likely to be valid. Accordingly, to treat these children simply with antidepressant medication is to focus on only a small, and possibly nonexistent, cause of their depression.

Addressing oneself to the more formidable environmental factors is the more reasonable approach even though it is a more difficult and complex undertaking and may not meet with much success.

Academic motivation is likely to be impaired in GMBDS children and this is not surprising. How can one expect an individual to be highly motivated in a situation in which there is predictable failure. Similarly, *academic curiosity* is compromised as they anticipate the failure that comes with the inability to understand what they are attempting to learn. And there are a variety of other secondary psychogenic manifestations that are beyond the scope of my presentation here. Some of the more common of these are listed in Table 2-1. Presumably, if the child did not suffer with the primary neurological manifestations, he or she would not exhibit the secondary psychogenic symptoms. This is not to say that these psychogenic symptoms cannot have other causes; rather, for these children the neurological impairments are the important (if not exclusive) contributing factors.

Psychogenic and/or Organic Symptoms

I now direct the reader to the items around the lower right segment of the largest circle in Figure 2-1, the section depicting symptoms that are psychogenic and/or organic. As can be seen from the diagram these are represented both inside and outside of the largest circle—indicating that I believe each of them to have both organic and psychogenic contributing factors. *Hyperactivity* is generally considered to be one of the cardinal signs of GMBDS, so much so that these children are sometimes referred to as *hyperactive children*— with the implication that this is the name of the disorder. I believe that there are some children who are genuinely hyperactive and who have been so from the intrauterine pe-

Table 2-1

COMMON SECONDARY PSYCHOGENIC MANIFESTATIONS OF THE GROUP OF MINIMAL BRAIN DYSFUNCTION SYNDROMES

Overly dependent for age
Frequent temper tantrums
Excessive silliness and
   clowning
Excessive demands for
   attention
Generally immature
Poor motivation
Takes path of least resistance
Ever trying to avoid
   responsibility
Poor follow-through
Low curiosity
Violent outbursts of rage
Cruelty to animals, children,
   and others
Destruction of property
Poor common sense in social
   situations
Very tense
Irritability, easily "flies off the
   handle"
Fears
   new situations
   being alone
   separation from parent
   school
   visiting other children's
   homes
   going away to camp
Disorganized
Depression
Low self-esteem

Little if any guilt over behavior
   that causes others pain
Little if any response to pun-
   ishment for antisocial
   behavior
Doesn't seek friendships
Rarely sought by peers
Not accepted by peer group
Doesn't respect the rights of
   others
Wanted things own way with
   exaggerated reaction if
   thwarted
Trouble putting self in other's
   position
Is often picked on and easily
   bullied by others
"Sore loser"
"Doesn't know when to
   stop"
Poor toleration of criticism
Little concern for personal ap-
   pearance or hygiene
Little concern for or pride in
   personal property
Withdrawn
Fears asserting self
Allows self to be easily taken
   advantage of
Gullible and/or naive
Passive and easily led
Excessive fantasizing, "lives
   in his(her) own world"

riod. Hyperactivity may exist in such pure form that no other primary neurological manifestations may be present. There are other children, however, in whom the hyperactivity appears to be part of the broader neurological picture and can justifiably be considered one of the primary neurological manifestations. However, hyperactivity can also be a concomitant of the tension that these children inevitably experience in the classroom. Because they are required to sit for hours in a classroom, where they may understand only a small fraction of what is being taught, they are likely to become edgy, fidgity, irritable, distractable, and agitated. As a result, they are likely to move around in and frequently get out of their seats, even though repeatedly warned not to do so. Their hyperactivity is a way of reducing the tension that is generated inevitably by their unfortunate situation. To consider the hyperactivity to be purely a neurological impairment is to take a narrow view of the symptom. It is best viewed as a composite of both a neurological predisposition and a concomitant of the tension that is generated in a classroom that will predictably cause tension, humiliation, and failure.

Much attention has been given to the *attentional deficit* of these children. The general consensus is that these children suffer with a neurologically based impairment in the capacity to sustain attention. The term *attention-deficit disorder* (*ADD*) is used by DSM-III (1980) to refer to this deficit. It is certainly the case that these children do not pay attention in the classroom. But who would under these circumstances? How can one continue to sustain attention in a situation where one doesn't understand a significant portion of what is being taught? In addition, attentional impairment is a concomitant of tension and anxiety, symptoms that these children inevitably exhibit in the classroom situation. Some claim that these children's attentional impairment is reasonably understood to be a manifestation of dysfunction in the alerting and arousal mechanisms of the brain (those mechanisms that must be supressed during sleep). They claim that the attentional impairment is a primary deficit in GMBDS children.

I believe that a pure *attention-deficit disorder* is extremely rare—so rare that for practical purposes it does not exist. The child with a pure attention-deficit disorder should have selective impairment on those subtests of the WISC-R (D. Wechsler, 1974) that specifically assess attentional capacity: Arithmetic, Digit Span, and Coding. Such a child should have normal or above average scores on the other nine subtests, those that are not so highly affected by the attentional factor. I have never seen such a child. I have seen, however, children who are depressed on so many of the subtests that they fall into the borderline or retarded intellectual range. These children, I agree, have an attention-deficit disorder; but they also have many other problems, problems that have resulted in their low scores on most of the other subtests. In fact, one can say that the alleged attentional deficit is the least of their problems—considering the fact that they have formidable difficulties with visual processing, auditory processing, and reasoning capacity. In Chapter Four of this book I will present in detail studies of mine which support my conclusion that there is no such clinical entity as an *attention-deficit disorder*.

Furthermore, the attentional deficit of ADD children is often diagnosed impressionistically and subjectively, without objective measurement criteria. A common scenario is for a teacher to make the diagnosis on the basis of her observation that the child is not paying as much attention as other children. She informs the parent of this problem and advises him or her to consult with a doctor. The pediatrician, child neurologist, or child psychiatrist who hears the story may not even observe the attentional impairment him- or herself, but out comes the prescription pad and the child is immediately placed on psychostimulant medication. And even the amount of medication is arrived at subjectively, a guess being made regarding what dosage level would be appropriate. The diagnosis is being made by hearsay and the treatment monitored by guesswork. It is reasonable to state that there are hundreds of thousands of children in the United States who are taking psychostimulant medication on an ongoing basis without any better evaluation than this. Because these children do not pay attention and because they are hyperactive they command significant attention in the classroom. It is for these reasons that the hyperactivity and attentional deficit have been given significant attention—more attention than these so-called impairments deserve. Children who interfere with the smooth flow of classroom routine are much more likely to gain the attention of their teachers than those who sit quietly, even though learning little or nothing. Because I consider hyperactivity and the attentional impairment to be minor factors in the difficulties of the GMBDS children (when one compares these deficits to their learning disabilities), I have relegated these symptoms to the small circles in the lower right segment of the largest circle in Figure 2-1.

I believe that GMBDS children's *impulsivity* has both neurophysiological and psychogenic components. These children have trouble "putting the brakes" on their thoughts and actions. I recall one GMBDS child who had a dream in which he was the engineer of a locomotive and he was unable to stop the train at each station. Rather, the train speeded past each stop as the prospective passengers on the platforms waved in frustration and fury as the train wizzed past them. Throughout the dream the engineer continually tried to stop the train by putting his foot on the brakes; but to no avail. The dream is an excellent statement of these children's inability to control voluntarily many of their actions. Impulsivity also has a cognitive component in that it involves forethought and planning. This is an important reason why many GMBDS children do poorly on the Mazes subtest of the WISC-R. These children also have difficulty projecting themselves into the future, whether it be the immediate or remote future. Not fully appreciating the future consequences of their acts, they are less likely to stop themselves from performing them. Besides these neurological contributions to impulsivity there are also, I believe, psychogenic factors. When an individual is operating under tension and stress (as is the case for these children in the classroom) impulsivity is likely to manifest itself. The edginess and jumpiness that contributes to their hyperactivity may also manifest itself as impulsivity. When one is tense one cannot "stop, look, and listen." One is too concerned with the sources of one's tension—in the case of these children the humiliations they anticipate with classmates, teachers, peers, siblings, their parents, and others.

I believe that the *disorganization* that these children manifest also has both neurological and psychogenic components. Psychologists know well that many of these children do poorly on the Block Design subtest of the WISC-R, in which the subject is asked to copy with colored blocks a pattern displayed on a sample card. Even under the most calm and placid conditions these children will often have difficulty performing this task. Poor performance on this subtest is generally attributed to neurologically based impairments in visual perception and/or eye-motor coordination. However, tension and anxiety are also likely to contribute to disorganization in that one is not likely to be able to concentrate on tasks when one is tense and anxious. Under such circumstances, one is less likely to be able to put things into proper sequence and arrange items within a pattern.

By *identification deficit* I refer to these children's impairment in their ability to project themselves into other people's situations. Those who work with these children will almost invariably remark on their impairments in providing sympathy (an intellectual process) and empathy (an emotional process). If there is one rule that these children have trouble following, it's the "golden rule." Lower animals have little if any capacity to do this (although animal lovers might disagree with me on this point). Whether or not lower animals can sympathize and empathize, there is no question that human beings are significantly superior with regard to this capacity (or at least some human beings). The ability to place oneself in another's position differentiates civilized human beings from uncivilized and primitive creatures, both human and nonhuman. I believe that these children's deficit in this area is partially the result of a neurophysiologically based cognitive impairment. Like many of the other deficits these children exhibit, the developmental element is very much operative here. Newborn infants cannot put themselves into other people's positions. The infant who bites the mother's breast does not appreciate that he or she is inflicting pain on the mother. As the child matures it becomes increasingly capable of such appreciation.

There are psychogenic factors, however, that contribute to these children's identification deficits. For a variety of reasons GMBDS children have few friends. They have difficulty understanding the rules of games. Concepts such as sportsmanship may completely confuse them. Their impulsivity, hyperactivity, and high level of tension interferes with their cooperating in games. They do not appreciate the subtleties of social nuances, facial expressions, and gestures. Because of the withdrawal their repertoire of information necessary for proper social functioning is limited. They are thereby deprived of learning about other people's feelings and placing themselves in other people's positions. This aspect of the identification problem is psychogenic and becomes added to the aforementioned neurophysiological element.

So much for the definition of the terms I will be using here. As mentioned, much unnecessary confusion has been introduced into this field by the lack of concensus regarding the definition of these terms. I do not claim to have proposed here final definitions, only those that seem reasonable to me and these will be the ones that I will be using in this book. At this point I will elaborate further on some of the phenomena discussed thus far in general terms only. Such descriptions will also provide further elaborations of the basic theory. In addition, in the course of these further elaborations I will define other terms that I use.

THE VISUAL PROCESSING DEFICITS

Table 2-2 depicts the various visual processing functions that one should consider when evaluating GMBDS children. The functions are presented in a sequence that goes from the most primitive (visual acuity) to the most sophisticated (visual language). Children with GMBDS do not generally exhibit impairments in the more primitive functions. These are the

Table 2-2

VISUAL PROCESSING

MINIMAL DIFFERENCES BETWEEN HIGHER APES AND HUMANS	ACUITY ATTENTION DISCRIMINATION	"SIMPLE"
MODERATE DIFFERENCES BETWEEN HIGHER APES AND HUMANS	GESTALT FIGURE-GROUND DISCRIMINATION	
FORMIDABLE DIFFERENCES BETWEEN HIGHER APES AND HUMANS	MEMORY ANALYSIS AND SYNTHESIS ORGANIZATION LANGUAGE	COMPLEX

functions in which there is little neuroanatomical difference between lower animals and human beings. As one progresses down the scale from the "simple" functions to the more complex, there is an increasing likelihood that GMBDS children will manifest symptomatology. This relates to the previously described theory that the greater the complexity of a function, the greater the likelihood that impairment will develop, and the less the likelihood that evolutionary selective processes will have stabilized the function.

Visual Acuity

I start with the "simplist" function, *visual acuity*. By visual acuity I refer simply to the ability to detect a visual stimulus, to ascertain whether or not something is being seen. It is only at the level at which an animal has eyes that one can meaningfully talk about visual acuity. It has nothing to do with the concept of the *meaning* or even identification of the visual stimulus, only whether or not a visual sensation is appreciated. GMBDS children rarely exhibit visual acuity deficits that play a significant role in their learning problems. Many optometrists would have us believe that this is not the case. The argument seems to go something like this: "One reads with one's eyes. Therefore, it is reasonable to say that if someone has trouble reading, it must be because of difficulties in the eyes." This is an absurd statement. It is true that one reads with one's eyes; but it is also true that one reads with one's brain. It is not simply the eyeballs that operate in the reading process. Rather, a whole network of neurological functions are involved and not simply the tracts that extend from the retinas back to the occipital cortices. The higher more complex visual association pathways are also involved. Therefore, any therapeutic program that directs its attention primarily to the eyeballs is not likely to have a significant effect on these children's learning disabilities. I am not saying that there are no

GMBDS children who may profit from ocular training; only that a small percentage have problems that warrant such treatment. In Chapter Eight of my book *The Objective Diagnosis of Minimal Brain Dysfunction* (1978b) there is a detailed discussion of this issue written by M. Schrier, an optometrist. My main point here is that the eyeballs of human beings and higher apes are practically identical, as are the tracts that extend from the retinas to the occipital cortices. Accordingly, on the basis of my theory, GMBDS children should have little difficulties in simple visual processes that involve the projection of visual stimuli from the outside world to the retina. And this is what I have found clinically. It would be an error for the reader to conclude that I am altering facts in order to fit my theory; rather, the theory has emerged from the observation that GMBDS children are not more likely to have problems in this area than children who are not in the GMBDS category.

Visual Attention

Visual attention, especially the capacity to sustain attention on a visual stimulus, is not, in my experience, generally impaired in GMBDS children. The statement, of course, contradicts prevailing notions about the so-called *attention-deficit disorder*. It may be that visual attention and auditory attention are separate functions. If so, I still hold with my previously discussed position that such an impairment does not exist in isolation from others. Furthermore, it is reasonable to assume that visual attention in humans is a primitive function which is similar in efficiency and stability to that of lower animals. After all, an animal that could not fix its eyes on a potential enemy was not likely to survive. Similarly, the animal that could not fix its eyes well on potential *prey* is also at a disadvantage for survival. The genes of animals with impairments in these areas have long ago been removed from the genetic pool.

objective instruments for assessing visual attention such as the Coding subtest of the WISC-R, the *Cancellation of Rapidly Recurring Target Figures Test* (R.D. Rudel et al., 1978) and the *Steadiness Tester* (R. Gardner et al., 1979) I have seen no evidence for *isolated* visual attentional deficits in children, whether normal or justifiably diagnosed as GMBDS. I generally only see such deficits in association with a wide variety of other neurologically based impairments and I suspect, even then, that the other functions assessed by the same instruments are more likely to be the cause of the low score than the visual attentional elements. For example, when a child does poorly on the Coding subtest of the WISC-R, I suspect that the primary reason for the poor performance is more likely a *memory impairment* or an *eye-hand motor coordination deficit*, than an attentional one. Deficits in either of the first two areas could explain a low score in the third, without postulating a specific deficiency in attention. In Chapters Three and Four I will discuss in further detail the studies that I have done that have led to my conclusion that GMBDS children generally do not suffer with an attentional deficit, visual or otherwise.

Visual Discrimination

By *visual discrimination* I refer to the capacity to differentiate between two visual stiumuli with regard to whether they are *the same* or *different*. A good example of a test that assesses such function is the one optometrists traditionally use to determine whether an individual is color blind. When administering this test, the patient is presented with an array of circles of varying hues, some of which are identical to one another and some of which are different from one another. Patients with normal eyesight will easily see a number that is formed by a series of circles that are of slightly different color from the surrounding ones. Patients with visual discrimination deficits have difficulty differentiating the numbers imbedded in the matrix of colored circles. Such "color blindness" is genetically determined and like eye color, skin color, and hair color, is not specifically correlated with the kinds of neurologically based deficits I am discussing here. My experience has been that very few GMBDS children have visual discrimination problems. Again, it is a primitive function related to the capacity to differentiate visually between animals that are friendly and those that are not, especially when the animals are very similar in appearance. Animals that could not make such differentiations were not as likely to survive as those that could. I suspect also that the neurological basis for this function is very similar in both human beings and lower animals.

The *Matching* subtest of this examiner's *Reversals Frequency Test* (R.A. Gardner, 1978a) assesses visual discrimination. The child is presented with a series of numbers or letters, each of which is followed by 4 renditions of the same number or letter, but presented in four different orientations. One orientation is the correct one, that is, it is identical to the model. The other 3 are not. The child is simply asked to encircle the one of the 4 that is identical to the model. GMBDS children rarely have difficulty with this test. Most often the scores of GMBDS children are within the normal range. In contrast, on the *Execution* subtest (in which they are asked to write a series of numbers and letters) and the *Recognition* subtest (in which they are asked to determine which one of a pair of mirror-image letters and numbers is correctly oriented and which is not) they generally do poorly. In my discussion of visual language (see below) I will discuss in detail the significance of the impaired performance of GMBDS children on these instruments. Similarly, as will be discussed below under *visual Gestalt*, GMBDS children are generally able to differentiate easily between correct copies of the model pictures presented to them and those that are incorrectly drawn (whether by themselves or others).

Visual Gestalt

Visual Gestalt refers to the capacity to envision a complete visual stimulus from one or a few of its component parts. The capacity for extrapolation is necessary here. For example, when shown a hand, the individual should be able to recognize that this is part of a complete human being—without actually being shown any other parts of the human body. Lower animals must be able to recognize that the observed paw of an enemy does not exist in isolation; but that behind the tree, bush, or other obstruction to a full view of what the paw may be connected to, there probably exists a total animal. The rabbit who sees only a wolf's tail extruding from behind a rock must be able to appreciate that connected to that tail there probably is a complete wolf with claws, a mouth, and teeth. Animals with *visual Gestalt* impairments did not survive over the course of evolution. Show a child a hand and a foot and it will generally recognize that these are parts of a person even though the other parts of the body are not shown.

L. Bender's *Visual Motor Gestalt Test* (1938 and 1946) is frequently used to detect children with GMBDS. I believe that these children's poor performance on this test is less related to an impairment in visual Gestalt then it is to a dyspraxia that interferes with their copying the forms presented to them. I use the word *dyspraxia* to refer to a disorder in which the hand does not appear to be able to follow the commands of the brain. Bona fide paralysis and coordination problems are not present in this disorder. It is as if there were some "blockage" between the pathways that connect those parts of the brain that initiate a cognitive command and those parts that send the final signals down the arm to produce hand movements. It is for this reason that the Geschwind (1965a, 1965b, 1971 and 1972) referred to this disorder as one type of "*dysconnexion syndrome.*" GMBDS children recognize well that they are not copying the Bender forms accurately, and they will differentiate easily between those copies that are correct and those that are inaccurate renditions. When asked why they therefore aren't copying what they see, they will reply that they have tried to but they can't.

Owen et al. (1971) conducted an excellent study that confirms this examiner's observations. Seventy-six learning-disabled (LD) and 76 academically normal children were administered the Bender Gestalt Test. After the test was over, each child was again shown every card and asked whether his or her copy was the same or different from the original. If different, the child was encouraged to discuss the exact ways in which his or her renditions were different. When the number of items scored as errors by the children were compared with the number of errors that the psychologists found, there was an overlap of 76% for accuracy of discrimination between the two groups. Not only were the LD children as good as the normals in identifying errors, but the agreement with the psychologists averaged about 75% for both groups.

The examiners then analyzed the 4 types of errors (distortion, rotation, integration, and perseveration) to determine the degree of agreement between the two groups of children as well as the psychologists who scored the tests. Of the 158 reproductions considered by the LD children and psychologists to have errors, 110 (69%) were judged to be the same type of error. The normal children had 114 agreements of errors with the psychologists, of which 76 (64.9%) were judged to be the same type of error. The difference between the 2 groups was not significant. In short, LD children were as accurate as normals in identifying the type of error made and both groups were in agreement with the psychologists on about 66% of the errors.

The authors conclude that it is not because of an impairment in "visual perception" that the LD children do more poorly than normals on the Bender Gestalt Test. Rather, they consider these children's problems to lie in two areas. They noted that many of their errors were related to improper *sequencing* of the material. In addition, they observed that many of the children had trouble *"constructing"* what they were trying to copy.

The Object Assembly subtest of the WISC-R also assesses visual Gestalt quite well. The subject is presented with an array of small wooden plaques of various sizes and shapes. The task is to put them together to form a complete figure (an animal, car, face, etc.). My experience has been that children with GMBDS often do have difficulty with the Object Assembly test and this problem, I believe, is related to difficulties in forming visual Gestalten. The reader cannot but be wondering at this point whether GMBDS children do or do not have problems in this area. The answer is related to the complexity of the task involving visual Gestalt functioning.

To elaborate, I believe that GMBDS children do not have visual Gestalt problems with regard to *simple* visual patterns such as recognizing that where there is a tail there must be a complete animal. Rather, any visual Gestalt problems they do exhibit are detected only in *complex* assessments of this function, tests that lower animals would not be expected to perform successfully. As mentioned, the poor performance of GMBDS children on Bender's *Visual Motor Gestalt* Test is more likely related to dyspraxia, than an impairment in visual Gestalt capacity. And I believe that the poor performance of GMBDS children on the Object Assembly subtest of the WISC-R is likely the result of impairments in visual organization capacity (a more complex function) and in visual Gestalt capacity for *complex* and subtle visual patterns. An automotive engineer might be able to envision the rest of a complex diagram of an automobile transmission system from visualization of only a small part. Or someone sophisticated with electronic diagrams might be able to extrapolate from a small section and appreciate the whole. GMBDS children, like higher apes, will have trouble with these more complex and sophisticated extrapolations.

Accordingly, I consider visual Gestalt capacity to represent a visual processing function that can be viewed as partway between the simpler and more primitive functions, which are not likely to be impaired in GMBDS children (like visual attention and visual discrimination), and the more complex visual processing functions, which are much more likely to be impaired (like visual memory and visual language). Therefore, GMBDS children will not generally have difficulties with the simpler tests of visual Gestalt, but do have problems with more complex tasks in this realm.

Visual Figure-Ground Discrimination

I use the term figure-ground discrimination to refer to the capacity to differentiate between more meaningful foreground visual stimuli and less meaningful background stimuli. Crucial here is the recognition that the foreground stimuli are more likely to be important than those in the background. We are dealing here with a function that is not simply one of *depth perception* but also of *meaning*. When we look at a scene we are not simply concerned with a two dimensional configuration. Although a visual display may have a two-dimensional representation on each of the retinas, our two eyes together enable us to appreciate depth. However, we must also have the ability to differentiate between important and unimportant aspects of the visual image. Sometimes the important element is in the foreground and sometimes in the background. The situation may require us to give special attention to this particular segment of the visual display.

Visual *figure-ground discrimination* impairment is not, in my opinion, frequently seen among MBD children. A.A.

Strauss and L. Lehtinen (1947) and A.A. Strauss and N.C. Kephart (1955), pioneers in this field, considered impairment in this area to be a primary deficit in the "brain-injured children" they described many years ago. Lower animals must have good figure-ground discrimination to detect their prey, especially when well camouflaged. They must be able to differentiate well between predatory animals that are close to them from threatening animals that are far away. Such differentiation is crucial in determining whether they will fight or flee. In addition, they must be able to detect potential predators when camouflaged. Such capacity has been of great survival value. Accordingly, I believe it is reasonable to conclude that animals with poor figure-ground discrimination were long ago killed off in the fight for survival.

I believe that GMBDS children do not generally have difficulty with *simpler* forms of figure-ground discrimination; but they do have problems with the more *complex* types that are to be found in sophisticated tests that assess this function — tests that assess at a level of complexity beyond that required of lower animals in the state of nature. Many GMBDS children have difficulty differentiating between complex geometric patterns imbedded in an array of other geometric forms. The *Southern California Perceptual-Motor Tests* (A.J. Ayres, 1968) and the *Figure-Ground Discrimination* subtest of the *Developmental Test of Visual Perception* (Frostig, 1961) are be good examples of instruments that assess this function in a way that is far more complex that would be required of lower animals in the state of nature. Accordingly, it is reasonable to say that some GMBDS children do exhibit impairments in this area, but their impairments do not relate to figure-ground tasks that are similar to an animal's determining whether another "background" animal in the jungle or woods is "friend or foe." They may have difficulty making figure-ground discriminations in complex cognitive tasks administered by a psychologists. Accordingly, I place figure-ground discrimination to be an example of visual processing in which there are moderate differences between higher apes and humans (Table 2-2).

Visual Memory

I use the term *visual memory* to refer to the capacity to store and retrieve information related to visual stimuli. The capacity to perform this function covers a whole range from the recall of visual stimuli that have just been introduced recently (short-term memory) to those that were experienced in the distant past (remote memory). Visual memory is the first of those functions in which the GMBDS child is likely to differ significantly from lower animals. A lower animal, if it is to survive, must remember the appearance of its foes and to have both short-term and long-term memory with regard to such visual imagery. It must have stored a visual image of a wide variety of other living forms and then *compare* these past images with those of present ones and then make decisions regarding whether or not fight or flight is in order. Human beings, as well, must be able to recall visual imagery related to both friends and foes if they are to function adequately and adapt in a competitive world. But the human being's visual memory goes far beyond this. The human is capable of performing prodigious tasks involving visual memory. There are individuals who have literally memorized the whole Bible. There are organic chemists who can recall at will dozens and even hundreds of pages of complex organic chemical formulas. There are electrical engineers who can recall hundreds of pages of complex electronic diagrams. A human being's capacity to memorize visual material can be truly awe inspiring. Actors routinely memorize thousands of lines in a script of a play. There is no lower animal that can come close to such an amazing capacity. This difference demonstrates well my position, stated so many times previously, that the greater the disparity between the human being and the higher ape with regard to a particular neurological function the greater the likelihood a GMBDS child will exhibit a deficiency in that function.

Visual Analysis and Synthesis

Visual analysis refers to the ability to break down a visual stimulus into its component parts and *visual synthesis* refers to the ability to build up a composite *visual pattern* from its component parts. Visual analysis and visual synthesis are complementary. The Block Design subtest of the WISC-R assesses this function. When administering this instrument, the subject is presented with an array of blocks with varying designs on the facets of each cube. The subject is asked to so arrange the cubes that they reproduce the pattern depicted on a card presented by the examiner. It is not likely that there is an analogy for this function among lower animals. The development and survival of modern technological societies are dependent upon the capacity of the humans to create and draw (synthesize) and understand (analyze) complex electronic, mechanical, and architectural diagrams. Even the most "brilliant" higher ape cannot be expected to perform such sophisticated functions. These functions are a very recent development on the evolutionary scale and therefore are more likely to be impaired in GMBDS children.

Visual Organization

Visual organization refers to the capacity to place the components of a visual array into their proper arrangement. This function is also assessed by the Block Design and Object Assembly subtests of the WISC-R. One must not only be able to identify the various components in the analytic process, but the synthetic process of building them up again involves the ability to place each component in its proper place in relation to the others. Building any complicated instrument such as an automobile, TV set, computer, etc. involves the capacity for visual organization. Again, this is not a function that lower animals have needed to develop to any significant degree. This is not to say that there are no analogies for this in lower animals. A beaver must be able to build a dam, ants build organized labrynthian colonies, and birds their nests. However, the organizational capacity necessary for these lower animals to perform these operations is relatively simple compared to the organizational capacity necessary for humans to function adequately in our complex technological society. Again, GMBDS children are likely to have impairments in organizational capacity because it is a function in which humans far surpass higher apes.

Visual Language

Visual Language, as previously discussed, refers to the ability to form a link or association between an entity and the visual symbol (word) that by social convention has been selected to denote the entity. It is only after years of training that a higher ape might be taught to "read" a few words, but it will never surpass the reading level of a bright 3- or four-year-old who is taught this function. There are human beings who can read in 35 different languages; perhaps a "genius" ape can be taught to "read" 35 words. I have placed the word "read" in quotes when using the term with apes because one cannot be certain about what the cognitive processes are inside the ape's head that enable it to perform a particular task after being presented a card on which is printed a word related to that task. It may be that a relatively simple conditioned reflex is operating here, and nothing more. If this is indeed the situation, then the word *read* may not be appropriate because of its implication of the presence of higher cognitive processes involving the appreciation of *meaning*. In short, then, it is in the area of reading that human beings are formidably different from lower animals and it is therefore in this area that GMBDS children are highly likely to have problems.

The term *dyslexia* is frequently used to refer to children who cannot read. This is another word which has become loosely defined in recent years. Most who use the word do not concern themselves with differentiating between reading disabilities that have a neurophysiological basis and those that are psychogenic. Some merely define dyslexia as a reading impairment in which the child is reading 2 years below the expected grade level for age, regardless of the cause. Included here then would be children who are behind in reading because of neurological deficit, those whose psychological problems have interfered with their reading capacity, as well as those whose educational systems have been inadequate. I prefer to confine the use of the word dyslexia to reading impairments related to neurophysiological deficits. A number of neurological factors may contribute, either alone or in combination, to a child's being dyslexic.

There may be a linguistic problem in which the child cannot properly link the visual symbol (word) with the entity which it has been designed to denote. There may be a problem in visual memory in which there is weakness of storage, so that the word does not get deeply entrenched in the neurological system. One can compare this to writing words in sand as opposed to writing words in concrete. Or there may be a problem in retrieval, i.e., the words are stored but the child cannot find the proper one at the proper time. It is as if the filing cards on which each word is written are not properly arranged in alphabetical order so that retrieval becomes chaotic. Teachers often refer to this phenomenon as "word finding." There may be a problem in appreciating the differences between correctly and incorrectly oriented numbers and letters. This is often referred to as a *reversals problem*. At the age of 1 or so, when a child first learns the meaning of the word "chair," differentiation is not generally made between chairs that face east and chairs that face west. A chair is a chair, regardless of its orientation. The same lack of concern for orientation is present with regard to the vast majority of other objects the child learns to identify. And orientation differentiations may not be made until the child starts to learn to read. Then, the teacher is generally going to point out to the child that the "b" is not the same as the "d," even though the figures are basically identical. This differentiation in orientation is a sophisticated consideration and may be a burden for children with neurological linguistic deficits. I consider a high frequency of reversal errors to be a good "marker" for the presence of dyslexia. When it is present, it is likely that the child will have difficulty reading, and it is likely, also, that some of the other aforementioned neurological deficits that contribute to dyslexia will also be present.

One of the problems for examiners in this field has been the vagueness of the criteria utilized to ascertain whether a child is truly exhibiting a high reversals frequency. Many examiners will simply ask a 6- or 7-year-old child to write a few sentences and if a letter appears that is incorrectly oriented, the examiner will conclude that the child is "dyslexic." No attempt is made to compare this child's reversals frequency to that of normal children. In order to rectify this deficit, the author has devised three *Reversals Frequency Tests* (R.A. Gardner, 1978a). Mention has already been made of this instrument in my discussion of visual discrimination, wherein I focused on the *Matching* subtest. Here I discuss in greater detail the other two reversals frequency tests because of their more specific relevance to the more complex factors involved in understanding and assessing visual language deficits. When administering the *Recognition* subtest the child is presented with pairs of letters and numbers. In each pair one item is correctly oriented and one is not. The child is simply asked to put a cross over the one of the 2 items that is "pointing in the wrong direction." Scores of normal children and those known to have neurologically based learning disabilities are provided, enabling the examiner to compare objectively the child being tested with others in each of these two categories. When administering the *Execution* subtest the child is asked to write a series of 1-digit numbers and lower case letters and the examiner merely scores the number of reversed items. These scores are compared with normals and those with known neurologically based learning disabilities, again enabling the examiner to compare objectively the child's scores with others in these 2 groups.

Although both of these instruments assess reversals frequency, they actually cover different areas of neurological functioning. In the *Recognition* subtest the child is merely being assessed for correct recall of whether the presented item is correctly or incorrectly oriented in accordance with the social convention for that particular item (letter or number). The child is not being asked to say anything about the underlying *meaning* of the item and what purpose it serves in the English language. Presumably an Oriental, with no previous experience with the English language, but who had the opportunity to peruse books, signs, and other reading material, might be able to do well on the test because of some recollection of the conventional orientation of the letter or number. When performing the tasks involved in the *Execution* subtest many more complex functions are called into operation. First, after hearing the item (letter or number) verbally presented by the examiner, the child must be able to retrieve from memory a visual image of that item. The child must then differentiate between correct and incorrect orientations of the retrieved item. The internal visual display of this item is then used as the model for copying it. A whole new series of operations are then called into play in order to execute this function. The child with *dyspraxia*, for example, might have a correct internal visual display but not be able to execute it because the hand does not seem to be able to follow the brain's commands. This child too might be called dyslexic. Although the *Execution* subtest assesses many more functions than the *Recognition* subtest, my experience has been that the *Recognition* subtest is the one of the 3 *Reversals Frequency Tests* that differentiates most sensitively dyslexic from normal children. The *Recognition* subtest, therefore, is the one that is the most sensitive for assessing the presence of a visual language deficit—a deficit that is likely to be seen in children with GMBDS because of the complexity and sophistication of the function and its relatively late appearance in human evolution.

THE AUDITORY PROCESSING DEFICITS

I discuss here the auditory processing deficits of GMBDS children, again in the sequence from the "simple" to the complex (Table 2-3). I place the word *simple* in quotation marks because these functions are certainly simple when compared to the more sophisticated and complex function of auditory language, but they are certainly not simple per se in that they are indeed highly complex and even marvelous functions.

Auditory Acuity

I use the term *auditory acuity* to refer simply to the capacity to hear. It is the simplest auditory function and, presumably, the first animals to have hearing organs were capable of utilizing this function. It does not refer to the capacity to give *meaning* to the auditory stimulus; only to the ability to ascertain whether or not an auditory stimulus is present and has been received. The traditional audiogram assesses this function in that all the patient need do is say whether or not a sound has been heard. Although GMBDS children may have hearing deficits it is not generally a primary cause or manifestation of GMBDS. There are a small percentage of GMBDS children,

Table 2-3

AUDITORY PROCESSING

MINIMAL DIFFERENCES BETWEEN HIGHER APES AND HUMANS	ACUITY ATTENTION DISCRIMINATION	"SIMPLE"
MODERATE DIFFERENCES BETWEEN HIGHER APES AND HUMANS	GESTALT FIGURE-GROUND DISCRIMINATION	
FORMIDABLE DIFFERENCES BETWEEN HIGHER APES AND HUMANS	MEMORY ANALYSIS AND SYNTHESIS ORGANIZATION LANGUAGE	COMPLEX

however, who I believe do develop more central auditory processing deficits as the result of middle ear infections in early childhood. It is not simply the middle ear and the inner ear that may be affected but, I believe, that such infections somehow extend themselves into the more central tracts involved in auditory processing. These children, however, represent a very small fraction of GMBDS children. Basically, GMBDS children have intact inner ears and normal auditory acuity.

Auditory Attention

I use the term *auditory attention* to refer to the ability to sustain concentration on an auditory stimulus. It may be that auditory and visual attention are separate functions. Lower animals must be able to sustain attention in the auditory realm if they are to survive. And they must be able to maintain such attention for long periods if they are to hear properly the sounds made by their enemies in the state of nature. When a rabbit hears a wolf's cry, it must "hang in there" and try to determine *over time* whether the wolves are coming closer or receding. This phenomenon is entirely separate from the rabbit's ability to *differentiate* the wolf's cry from other sounds and to *recognize* the meaning of the wolf's cry as a dangerous auditory stimulus. Animals with poor auditory attentional apparatus, then, were not as likely to have survived over the span of evolution.

Contrary to prevalant notions in child psychiatry at this point, I do not believe that most GMBDS children suffer with an isolated auditory attentional problem. To do so they would have to exhibit selective impairment on the 2 subtests of the WISC-R that are particularly sensitive to auditory attention, namely, Arithmetic and Digit Span. Certainly, children with low IQs may exhibit deficits on these two subtests, but they also have deficits in many other subtests—so much so that any purely auditory attentional problems they may have may be viewed as the least of their problems. A child with a pure auditory attentional deficit would have to have low scores on these 2 subtests *only* and be normal or average on the remaining. I have not seen such a child, nor have I seen children who exhibit isolated defects on other tests of auditory function that I myself have devised, namely, the *Word Span Test* and the *Compliance with Serial Verbal Instructions* test (These tests will be discussed in further detail in Chapters Three and Four). Again, when children do exhibit low scores on these instruments, they generally manifest deficiencies in a wide variety of other areas. Perhaps their attentional impairment is one of many impairments; perhaps other impairments are so formidable that other deficiencies, rather than the attentional, have produced low scores on these assessment instruments. The more reasonable explanation, I believe, and the one that is more consistent with the theory being presented here, is that an isolated attentional deficit does not exist in human beings.

Auditory Discrimination

I use the word *auditory discrimination* to refer to the ability to differentiate between two auditory stimuli as to whether they are the *same* or *different*. It does not refer to the *meaning* of the sound. Understanding the meaning of a sound would justifiably be considered an auditory language function (which will be discussed below). A mother deer, while protecting her sleeping young at night, is likely to be awakened by the cries of a distant wolf; but may remain sleeping when exposed to the louder sound of an owl in the tree overhead. She must be able to differentiate precisely between the sounds of friendly animals and the sounds of enemies. Of course, auditory meaning comes into play here. I am not focusing here on this aspect of the deer's differentiation (but will do so on the section on *auditory language*). Rather, I am focusing only on the mother deer's ability to appreciate the *difference* between the sound of the wolf and the sound of the owl. In addition, she must obviously be able to give an interpretation to the 2 sounds, to appreciate that the wolf's sound is a dangerous one and the owl's is not. Both functions are necessary for survival. Animals that could not make these differentiations were not likely to survive.

The *Auditory Discrimination Test* (J.M. Wepman, 1973) assesses this function. When utilizing this instrument, the child is presented with a series of paired words. Sometimes the 2 words are identical (house, house). Sometimes they sound alike but are different (book, brook). The child is merely asked to say whether the words are the same or different. The child is not asked any questions about recognition of the meaning of the words. Presumably, an Oriental child, with no familiarity whatsoever with the English language, could accomplish successfully these tasks. My experience has been that GMBDS children rarely have problems with this instrument. This is consistent with the theory presented here that this primitive function is not likely to be impaired in GMBDS children.

Auditory Gestalt

Auditory Gestalt refers to the ability to recognize a whole auditory stimulus from a part. It is certainly easy to see examples of this phenomenon in human begins. Musicians, for example, may be able to recognize a whole symphony from a few themes, or even a few notes. In normal human conversation we may miss part of a word but we can often extrapolate from the phonetic fragments that have been heard and appreciate the whole word that has been spoken. We also miss occasional spoken words, but surmise the meaning of what the speaker is saying from the other sentence components. Here too a kind of part-whole extrapolation is taking place. It is more difficult to envision an analogy in nature, but I suspect that there probably are. Animals are certainly sensitive to the sounds of other animals with regard to their *quality* in order to differentiate friend from foe. But this is basically a manifestation of auditory linguistic capacity, that is, the ability to give *meaning* to an auditory stimulus. Perhaps an animal can extrapolate from a single part of an auditory stimulus and respond to it as if the whole were presented. Perhaps a part of a mating call is enough to elicit the total mating response. Perhaps hearing a fraction of the danger sound, the beginning of a snake's hiss for example, might be enough for an animal to conclude what the rest of the sounds will be.

The *Illinois Test of Psycholinguistic Abilities* (ITPA) (S.A. Kirk et al., 1968) includes two tests that assess auditory Gestalt: Auditory Closure and Sound Blending. In the Auditory Closure subtest, the subject is presented with a word that is broken down into its phonetic components. However, one phonetic component is *omitted* and the subject is asked to ascertain the whole word. In Sound Blending the word is similarly presented in such a way that it is broken up into its phonetic components. However, here *all* the phonetic components are presented and the subject is asked to fuse them together and verbalize the proper pronouniciation. My experience has been that GMBDS children will occasionally have difficulty with these instruments. However, these are highly sophisticated auditory Gestalt functions and should be considered the kinds of auditory Gestalt tasks that relate to language and not the kinds that one finds in the state of nature in lower animals. It is for this reason that I place auditory Gestalt difficulties in the intermediate category of auditory processing, that category in which there are moderate differences between higher apes and humans.

Auditory Figure-Ground Discrimination

Auditory Figure-Ground Discrimination refers to the capacity to discriminate between auditory stimuli that are close and/or important from those that are distant and/or unimportant. The aforementioned mother deer must recognize that the loud voice of the owl in the nearby tree, although the more compelling stimulus, is not dangerous; whereas the distant sound of the wolf's howl, although of lower intensity, is the more important. Whereas previously I have referred to the auditory discrimination (owl's sound vs. wolf's sound) and auditory language (innocuous vs. dangerous) functions being considered in this vignette, I refer here to a third function, namely, the ability to ascertain whether the sound is close by or remote. Another animal function in the figure-ground category under consideration here is the ability to detect the sound of a foe when competing with other sounds that are neutral or those of friendly animals. For example, a jungle is filled with sounds. An animal must be able to distinguish the hiss of a snake from the surrounding chatter of monkeys, even though the monkeys' sounds may be far louder. Animals who are weak with regard to these figure-ground functions were less likely to survive over the span of evolution.

In human beings this capacity refers to the ability to differentiate important from unimportant auditory stimuli that impinge upon us. In a crowded room we generally can attend to the voice of the person to whom we are speaking and ignore the extraneous noise of other people's voices. The *Goldman-Fristoe-Woodcock Auditory Selective Attention Test* (1974) assesses this function. Here the child is presented with a primary auditory stimulus in association with a variety of other increasingly competing sounds (fan and cafeteria noises). The competing noises becomes progressively louder, to the point where they drown out the primary stimulus. The instrument enables the examiner to assess objectively the child's capacity to "hang in" with the primary stimulus. My experience has been that some GMBDS children have trouble with this test. However, it assesses primarily *linguistic* figure-ground discrimination, a highly human function. It does not assess the more primitive kinds of auditory figure-ground discrimination seen in lower animals. The occasional impairment of GMBDS children in this area fits in well with the theory being proposed here, that figure-ground discrimination is an intermediary function on the evolutionary scale and that GMBDS children should have difficulties on the more sophisticated, typically human, tasks, but not on the more primitive ones.

Auditory Memory

Auditory Memory refers to the ability to store and retrieve information derived from auditory stimuli. This is the first of the more complex functions under consideration here, the ones in which the human being differs significantly from the higher apes. Lower animals are certainly able to recall simple auditory commands (dogs remember their names) but their memory for complex auditory messages is far less sophisticated than that of human beings. There are people who can train themselves to repeat in correct sequence 60 to 70 numerals presented to them only once. The Digit Span subtest of the

WISC-R assesses short-term auditory memory. The patient is presented with progressively longer series of single-digit numbers and asked to repeat them (first forward and then backward) in the exact order presented by the examiner. As mentioned, my experience has been that children with GMBDS rarely exhibit an isolated impairment on this subtest. This is related, I believe, to the fact that they do not generally suffer with a pure attention-deficit disorder. However, when they do have difficulty with this instrument, they generally have problems with many of the other subtests of the WISC-R as well. The reason for this, I believe, is that they have other more formidable cognitive impairments, only one of which is in auditory memory. It is this·impairment, more than the attentional, that interferes with their functioning on the Digit Span subtest.

Auditory Analysis and Synthesis

Auditory analysis refers to the ability to break down an auditory stimulus into its component parts. Auditory synthesis, its opposite, refers to the process by which component parts are formulated into a composite structure. An example of auditory analysis and synthesis would be the ability to break down a word into its phonetic components and then reconstruct it back into the original word. The Sound Blending subtest of the ITPA assesses this kind of auditory synthesis. Another example is the ability to break down a sentence or paragraph into its composite parts and then rebuild it. The same process can be applied to a piece of music.

It is difficult to imagine lower animals, or even higher apes, performing this function to a significant degree. It is a highly sophisticated process that is clearly a very recent development on the evolutionary scale. Even if higher apes can be taught to perform such functions, their capacity to do so is clearly far inferior to that of the human being, even the human child. Consistent with the theory being proposed here, it is not surprising that children with GMBDS often exhibit problems utilizing these processes.

Auditory Organization

Auditory organization refers to the ability to organize auditory stimuli into a proper and reasonable arrangement. It is related to the ability to analyze and synthesize auditory stimuli. When writing music one must appreciate certain patterns and put them in a particular order. Lower animals cannot write symphonies. When listening to a speech, full understanding includes the ability to place the various parts in proper perspective and to consider a hierachy of significance and importance. Lower animals cannot join debating teams, function as courtoom litigators, become theatre critics and write reviews of plays, or otherwise perform functions that rely upon the capacity to organize meaningfully auditory stimuli. GMBDS children are likely to have problems in this area to a significant degree. This deficiency plays a role in their "not listening " to their parents. When the parents of these children say, "He doesn't listen to me," they are often referring to the inability of the child to perform in proper order a sequence of requests. Most parents of GMBDS children know better than to say to such a child: "When you get home from school, change into your play clothes, play for an hour, then do some homework, then wash your hands, then we'll have supper, and then you can watch television for an hour." This impairment is not simply due to attentional deficit (if there be one present) and/or memory impairment (often present). Compromised ability to organize auditory stimuli may also play a role.

Auditory Language

Auditory Language is the most sophisticated and advanced auditory processing function. As mentioned, auditory linguistic capacity refers to the ability to appreciate an association between an entity and the auditory stimulus (word) that society, by convention, has agreed will denote it. Although higher apes can be taught to "understand" and respond to simple words, they are generally no match for the average toddler. There are people who can understand 35 languages. Not surprisingly, GMBDS children often exhibit difficulties in this area. It is the most highly complex and sophisticated of the auditory processing functions and is quite commonly impaired in GMBDS. When GMBDS children have difficulty paying attention in school, I believe that it is more likely related to a weakness in auditory linguistic capacity than it is to a basic inability to sustain attention. Rather, because these children often have a primary impairment in processing auditory linguistic stimuli, they do not understand well what the teacher is saying. Accordingly, they become restless and inattentive — behavior which becomes labeled "hyperactivity" and/or "attention-deficit disorder." I believe that if these children were able to understand better what the teacher was saying, they would be less frustrated, impulsive, and hyperactive. They would pay attention for longer periods because they would be able to comprehend what is being said.

LOGICAL REASONING DEFICITS

The impairments in logical reasoning that GMBDS children frequently exhibit are not generally given the attention they deserve. Yet, these impairments are often formidable and are likely to play a significant role in their deficiencies in the classroom, in the neighborhood, and at home. As can be seen from Figure 2-1 the reasoning deficits, along with the visual processing and auditory processing deficits, comprise the neurologically based learning disabilities.

Reasoning impairments are a central element in these children's inability to attend to what the teacher is saying. Not understanding what is being taught, they become inattentive. Differentiation must be made between linguistic problems and reasoning problems. Reasoning problems may be viewed partially as a subdivision of linguistic problems. They represent, in part, the impairment in utilizing more sophisticated types of linguistic material. For example, a child with a simple linguistic problem may have trouble associating the written word "book" with the entity which that visual symbol has been designed to denote. The process is a relatively concrete one in which the visual symbol (the word) is designed to denote an actual concrete object (the book). Reasoning deficits refer to more sophisticated utilization of language. For example, the word *independence* has no concrete representation. It is an abstraction. GMBDS children are more likely to have difficulty with such words. At an even higher level, they have trouble with complex abstractions and conceptualizations — those involved, for example, in doing arithmetic computations. And the more abstract the processes, the more difficulty GMBDS children are likely to have. The same problems interfere with their understanding the rules of games and the concept of sportsmanship, and these impairments interfere with their ability to make friends.

The *Columbia Mental Maturity Scale* (B.B. Burgemeister et al., 1972) is an excellent instrument for assessing the child's capacity for inductive logic and visual conceptualization. The child is presented with a series of plates on each of which is a linear array of pictures. In the simplest examples, one picture does not belong with the other 4. In the more complex presentations of the 5 pictures, 2 form one set, 2 form another set, and the 5th belongs to neither set. The child is simply asked which picture does not belong with the others. It is a very attractive instrument and most children rise to the challenge of identifying the picture that does not belong with the others.

The Similarities subtest of the WISC-R is also useful in assessing logical reasoning capacity. The child is presented with a series of paired words and asked to describe how they are alike, for example, "How are an apple and a banana alike?" One point credit is given for responses that are correct, but at a more concrete level ("You can eat them both"). Two points credit are given for more abstract responses ("They're both fruits"). The instrument assesses analagous logic, auditory conceptualization, and abstraction capacity. The Arithmetic subtest of the WISC-R is also a useful instrument for assessing objectively logical reasoning capacity. The child is presented with progressively more difficult arithmetic problems. Younger children start with a few simple visual problems (counting the number of trees), but older children are administered primarily verbal questions, for example, "A boy had 12 newspapers and sold 5. How many did he have left?" The instrument assesses arithmetic logic, concentration, auditory and visual conceptualization, and abstraction capacity.

The capacity to understand verbal analogies is generally considered to be highly correlated with one's logical reasoning capacity. The *Scholastic Aptitude Test* (SAT), taken by high school students planning to go on to college, is based on this assumption. A verbal analogies typical question: "Butter is to bread as X is to tea." (Sugar would be a possible correct answer.) The Verbal Reasoning subtest of the *Differential Aptitude Tests* (G.K. Bennett et al., 1974) assesses well the child's capacity to understand and formulate verbal analogies.

As indicated on Figure 2-1, I designate the visual processing deficits, auditory processing deficits, and logical reasoning deficits to comprise the three major components of the entity which I refer to as the *neurologically based learning disabilities*. Of the 5 areas in which we differ significantly from higher apes, these are the 3 that are most likely to interfere with the child's learning in school. Although the soft neurological signs and speech deficits (see below) are also areas of impairment in these children, they are less likely to interfere directly with the learning process. Accordingly, I do not classify them among the neurologically based learning disabilities.

SOFT NEUROLOGICAL SIGNS

In a sense, every sign described in this book could justifiably be called a soft neurological sign. The group of minimal brain dysfunction syndromes, by definition, is a collection of mild neurological syndromes (still to be clearly delineated from one another) that share in common varying degrees of minimal, but definite, neurological impairment. At this time, however, a certain subgroup of GMBDS is referred to by the term soft neurological signs. Because of the widespread use of the term I will also subscribe to the convention, but recognize that the term is a poor one and that we do better to describe more specifically each of the entities subsumed under the rubric than to artificially pull together certain clusters as if the members had a certain special relationship.

Table 2-4

SOFT NEUROLOGICAL SIGNS

MOTOR DEVELOPMENTAL LAGS

REFLEX ABNORMALITIES
(↑, ↓, AND OVERFLOW)

MOTOR IMPERSISTENCE

COORDINATION DEFICITS

TREMORS AND CHOREIFORM MOVEMENTS

DYSPRAXIAS

The term soft neurological signs was, to the best of my knowledge, first introduced by L. Bender (1947) in a discussion of minor neurological impairments seen in children with schizophrenia. Many, such as T. Ingram (1973), do not believe in the existence of such signs and consider use of the term a manifestation of "soft thinking" on the part of those examiners who believe in the concept. R.J. Schain (1975) is also dubious about the existence of soft neurological signs because of the vague criteria upon which they are often based and low interexaminer agreement found when multiple examinations of the same patient are conducted. These drawbacks to identification notwithstanding, I personally am an adherent to the concept. It seems reasonable to me that for many signs and symptoms there should be borderline and intermediate states, rather than just a present or absent situation. The best way to settle this conflict is to conduct objective studies of both normals and those with GMBDS, in which one *quantifies* the findings. In many areas such data are already available and have been presented by the author in great detail elsewhere (R.A. Gardner, 1979) and readily confirm the existence of such intermediate states. For many other soft neurological signs, studies still need to be done to determine whether or not they in fact do exist. The central problem facing those who would try to define such signs is where to draw the line that demarcates the normal from the abnormal. Let us say that in a given population the average male's height is 5 ft. 6 in. At what point does one say that a male is "short"? Does one use 5 ft. 1 in., 4 ft. 10 in., 3 ft. 8 in., or any other particular height? Similarly, what cut-off point does one use to define a person as "tall"? Clearly, such points of differentiation are arbitrary. The best solution to this probelm is to present a value in terms of *standard deviation from the mean or percentile rank*. With such data examiners can decide for themselves what significance they wish to ascribe to the data: how many standard deviations from the mean or what percentile rank warrants a particular label. Accordingly, the examiner can state, for example, "Robert can stand longer on one foot than 90% of boys his age" or "The age at which Jane began to walk is later by 2 standard deviations than the average for girls."

The soft neurological signs do not lend themselves well to being divided into a continuum from the most primitive to the most sophisticated. Table 2-4 lists what I consider to be the most common forms of soft neurological signs. Many are well viewed to be the result of weaknesses in complex neurological functions that are lately developed on the evolutionary scale.

Motor Developmental Lags

Children with *Motor Developmental Lags* are late with respect to the ages at which they reach the various developmental milestones. These symptoms are manifestations of developmental lags such as lateness in suppressing such primitive signs as the Babinski and tonic neck reflexes; significiant lateness in such developmental milestones as standing, walking, talking, and bowel and bladder training; and persistence of immature speech patterns on a neurological (as opposed to a psychogenic) basis. In order to detect their presence such signs have to be elicited during the period in which they should have disappeared, but *before* they belatedly do so. For example, the average child begins to walk during the 10-14 month period. A child who is still not walking at 19 months would be considered by most examiners to have a neurological developmental lag that many would label a soft neurological sign. If at 20 months the child begins to walk, the sign would not longer be present. If the child was first seen at 20 months then one would have to make some judgment about the parents' reliability in order to decide whether or not such a sign was present. (Signs, by definition, are manifestations observed by the examiner.) This introduces a subjective element at times which may compromise the credibility of those who report such signs. However, a small percentage of those who develop late may still exhibit mild neuromuscular or neurophysiological problems in walking. They may be clumsy, have difficulty running, and show other manifestations of gross and/or fine motor coordination deficits.

Nerve cell myelinization provides *one example* of the way in which the developmental type of soft neurological sign may be brought about. P. Yakovlev and A. Lecours (1967), in an excellent study, have demonstrated that there is great variation among the parts of the brain with regard to the age when myelinization is completed. Myelinization begins during fetal life and terminates at different times in different parts of the brain. Although most nerve fibers in the brain are completely myelinated by the third to fourth year of life, certain sections of the brain do not complete the process until many years later. The reticular formation, for example, is not fully myelinated until the teens and many intercortical association fibers only complete the process *during the fourth decade of life*. It is reasonable to assume that nerve fibers do not function optimally until completely myelinated and that children whose myelinization is particularly slow will manifest various types of neurological immaturity. Some children with such developmental lags may only represent the lower end of the bell-shaped curve for myelinization rate. In others, disease processes may have caused the retarded myelin development and exposure to detrimental extrinsic influences may bring about developmental lag. It would be an error for the reader to conclude that *all* children with such developmental lags have symptoms that are the result of such myelinization impairment. In all probability far more complex factors are involved and the myelinization example has been presented to provide a concept and/or a theory of explanation for what is probably applicable to only a small percentage of all GMBDS children.

Reflex Abnormalities

By *Reflex Abnormalities* I refer here only to such abnormalities as hyperreflexia, hyporeflexia, and motor spread (or overflow). The latter refers to the phenomenon in which, for example, a knee-jerk is elicited and instead of the knee only reacting reflexly the whole lower extremity does. In more extreme cases the other knee will reflexly jerk as well, so massive is the overflow reaction. Another example would be a broadening of the area from which the Babinski reflex can be elicited. Normally, it is present at birth and, at that time, can be elicited from a wide area: not simply from the stimulation of the soles of the foot, but the legs, thighs, and even the lower abdomen. As the child grows older, the area from which the reflex can be elicited progressively shrinks. Finally, by 20 months of age, or so, it can be only elicited by stimulating the dorsal or solar aspects of the foot and by 24 months of age the reflex disappears entirely (W. Brain and M. Wilkinson, 1959). Children with neurodevelopmental lags will exhibit Babinski responses from areas broader than those that would be expected at that particular age. For example, a 20-month-old with such a lag might exhibit the response from stimulation of the thighs. In addition, during the period when the reflex is becoming obliterated, there are times when it may be elicited and times when it may not be. The only thing that one can say with certainty is that by 24 months it should no longer be present and that children who exhibit it beyond that time are strongly suspect for neurological dysfunction.

Motor Impersistence

Younger children cannot maintain a state of muscle contraction as long as older children. For example, they cannot stand on one foot, clench their fists or keep their eyes shut as long as older ones. There is a developmental progression of the capacity to maintain muscle tension on a voluntary basis and children with GMBDS may exhibit lags in such progression. The term *motor impersistence* was first used by M. Fisher (1956) to refer to the impairment in this function. The phenomenon was defined by J.C. Garfield et al. (1966) as the "inability to sustain certain voluntary motor acts initiated on verbal command." They considered the impairment to be the result of a primary defect in sustaining attention. A.L. Benton (1970) subsequently used the following definition: "the inability to sustain an act that has been initiated on command." Elsewhere (R.A. Gardner, 1979) I describe a series of tests that assess objectively this function (standing on one foot, keeping the eyes closed, protruding the tongue, and keeping the mouth open). In addition, the Steadiness Tester (R.A. Gardner et al., 1979) also assesses motor impersistence as well as other functions.

Coordination Deficits

Coordination Deficits refer to both fine and gross motor coordination difficulties. Examples of fine motor coordination difficulties would be problems in writing, playing the piano, typing, tying shoelaces, and serially opposing the tip of the thumb to the tips of the other four fingers. Examples of gross motor coordination deficits would be problems in running, throwing, catching, and walking. Of the various kinds of soft neurological signs, the coordination deficits are probably the ones that are of most significance with regard to the theory I am presenting here. As mentioned, this is the function that enables man to perform the kinds of complex manipulations that are necessary for the development and survival of our modern technological society. This is one of the important areas in which human beings differ formidably from even the highest ape. An ape may throw a rock and possibly wield a club in primitive fashion, but the ape cannot be taught to repair a fine watch. Not surprisingly, the areas of the human brain devoted to this function are massive compared to that of even the higher ape. Specifically, the area of the anterior parietal lobe devoted to motor innervation of the hand is enormous compared to the similar area in the ape's brain. The same is true of the hand's sensory area on the posterior part of the frontal lobe when one compares it with the similar area in the higher ape. With such formidable representation, it is not surprising that errors will occur on a chance basis with the result that certain children are likely to have weaknesses in their fine motor coordination functioning. These are the children we label GMBDS.

Tremors and Choreiform Movements

S. Brock (1945) defines a tremor as a "regular rhythmic, alternating contraction of muscle group or groups and their antagonists." Tremors are generally considered to be a manifestation of disease of the basal ganglia. R. Paine and T. Oppé (1966) describe two categories of tremors: fine and course. Fine tremors are generally of 9-10/sec frequency. They may be familial in origin and may be seen in hyperthyroidism. Course tremors are slower, 3-5/sec, and may be seen with other manifestations of basal ganglia disease such as chorea, athetosis, dystonia, and hemiballismus. According to Paine and Oppé, if a tremor is not of one of the aforementioned frequencies, it cannot justifiably be referred to as a tremor, and psychogenic etiology or other disorder must be considered. Tremors are generally detected by observing the child's outstretched hands. Course tremors may be observed this way, but fine tremors may not so readily be seen. This is especially the case when the tremors are mild. In such cases electromyographic (EMG) studies may be useful in determining whether the child has tremors.

Chorea is defined by S. Brock (1945) as "brief, explosive, unsustained, abrupt movements, possessing a coordination comparable to that seen in voluntary movement." Unlike tremors, they do not have a fixed frequency; rather they are aperiodic. Brock describes them as "subjectively purposeful, but objectively aimless," i.e., the patient may attempt to rationalize them as having a function in order to deny their involuntary nature. Chorea is also the result of basal ganglia disease. Children with GMBDS sometimes exhibit mild chorea movements that are often referred to as choreiform movements. H.F.R. Prechtl and J. Stemmer (1962) consider such movements to be an important factor in hyperactive behavior. However, they do not present any evidence regarding the exact percentage of hyperactive children they consider to be excessively active because of choreiform movements. Tremors and choreiform movements are not too common among GMBDS children, in my experience. However, there are some who do exhibit such manifestations and they are generally the result of extrapyramidal and/or cerebellar impairment. My experience has been that when these symptoms are present the child usually has more severe problems than the average child who is diagnosed as GMBDS. Rather, they are more likely to be classified in the group of cerebral palsied children.

Dyspraxia

Dyspraxia is a more complex type of soft neurological sign. Here there is no basic motor or coordination problem. Rather, the extremity does not seem to be able to carry out the instructions of the brain. The person knows exactly what he or she wants to do, but the hand, for example, will not follow the brain's directions. This is what N. Geschwind (1965a, 1965b, 1971 and 1972) referred to as a "dysconnexion syndrome." It is as if there is a blockage of the connections between the cognitive centers of the brain (which direct the hands to perform the act) and the hand (specifically with regard to its capacity to follow the brain's instructions). The individual is completely aware that the hand is not doing what the brain wants it to do. Poor hand writing may be a manifestation of dyspraxia. As mentioned, children who do poorly on the Bender's *Visual Motor Gestalt Test* generally do so because of dyspraxia rather than the inability to perceive properly the geometric forms they are copying.

SPEECH DEFECTS

As mentioned, it is important to differentiate between *speech defects* and *language defects*. Speech refers to articulation whereas language refers to the ability to form an association between an entity and a visual symbol (written word) or auditory symbol (spoken word) which has by social convention been designed to denote that entity. The articulatory apparatus is found primarily in the pharynx and larynx. Centrally, the speech area of the brain has formidable representation when compared to the area devoted to speech functioning in lower animals. This is not surprising considering the capacity of the human being to articulate meaningfully hundreds of different languages. And, as mentioned, there are individuals who can speak in as many as 35. Because of the great variability of speech development among normal children, a child's level of speech maturation may be a poor criterion upon which to base a diagnosis of GMBDS (M. Charlton, 1973). In addition, psychological factors play an immensely important role in determining the rate at which children will learn to speak and the level of maturity they will attain. G. Wyatt (1969) and K. de Hirsch (1974) have emphasized how the mother's feedback, her availability as a speech model, and her involvement with the child play a vital role in speech development. Furthermore, regression of speech and fixation at immature speech levels are common manifestations of psychogenic disorders of childhood. Accordingly, delineating the purely neurological factors in abnormal speech development may be especially difficult. Yet, there are normal sequences of speech development that are neurologically based, and it behooves the examiner to be familiar with them if he or she is to properly evaluate the child with GMBDS.

Considering the massive complexity of the articulatory apparatus, it is reasonable that a certain percentage of individuals will have deficits that are purely related to the chance occurrence of malfunctioning neurons. Probably the two most common types of speech deficits that are manifestations of the kinds of problems I am referring to here are stuttering and lisping.

FURTHER COMMENTS ON PSYCHOGENIC LEARNING DISABILITIES

I have presented here a generalized statement of my views on the etiology and clinical manifestations of the GMBDS complex. The reader who is interested in more information on the clinical symptomatology (especially with regard to their objective diagnosis) does well to refer to my *The Object of Diagnosis of Minimal Brain Dysfunction* (1979). I have presented, as well, some of the more common secondary psychogenic symptoms. Table 2-1 lists what I consider to be other secondary psychogenic symptoms that are seen in GMBDS children. More details about the manifestations and treatment of these symptoms will be discussed in a forthcoming book tentatively entitled *Psychotherapy of the Psychogenic Problems of Children with Neurologically Based Learning Disabilities.*

It is important for the reader to differentiate between the psychogenic problems that are *secondary* to the organic/neurophysiological problems focused on in this presentation from the *purely psychogenic* learning disabilities. I have divided these into two categories: The *Primary Psychogenic Learning Disabilities* (Table 2-5) are those psychogenic learning problems that are direct manifestations of psychological problems related to school attendance and learning. The *Secondary Psychogenic Learning Disabilities* (Table 2-6) are those learning problems that are not etiologically school related. Rather, they are the result of psychological difficulties that stem from nonschool sources (especially the home). However, they tend to "spill over" into the learning area and so the child has difficulties in school as well as in the original areas of dysfunction. Again, it is beyond the scope of this article to discuss these in detail. These will, however, be discussed in a forthcoming book, tentatively entitled *The Diagnosis and Treatment of Psychogenic Learning Disabilities*.

Table 2-5

PRIMARY PSYCHOGENIC LEARNING DISABILITIES

IMPAIRED ACADEMIC MOTIVATION

IMPAIRED INTELLECTUAL CURIOSITY

ANTI-INTELLECTUAL ATTITUDE

ANTI-AUTHORITY ATTITUDE

SCHOOL CONDUCT DISORDER

SCHOOL REFUSAL

TRUANCY

SEPARATION ANXIETY DISORDER
("SCHOOL-PHOBIA")

INTELLECTUAL INHIBITIONS
("LEARNING BLOCK")

Table 2-6

SECONDARY PSYCHOGENIC LEARNING DISABILITIES

The wide variety of psychogenic disorders that can interfere with learning, e.g.

> Depression
> Compulsions
> Emotional inhibition
> Passive-dependency
> Passive-aggressivity
> Tension
> Fears
> Anxiety
> Obsessive preoccupation
> Psychosomatic disorders
> Withdrawal, especially autistic
> Hallucinations

IMPLICATIONS OF THE THEORY

Although I will be devoting relatively little space here to the implications of this theory, this should not be interpreted by the reader to mean that they are inconsequential or limited. Rather, the theory, if it is correct, has profound implications but only warrants little space for their description because they can be so simply stated.

First, the implications for the field of education are formidable. If I am correct, then educators and mental health professionals are labeling a phenomenon a disease process, when, in fact, we are only dealing with a normal segment of the population—a segment that is approximately at the 10-25th percentile levels of functioning in a variety of cognitive capacities. Furthermore, many professionals working with GMBDS children are operating under the assumption that these children can be brought up to normal levels and that concerted efforts should be utilized to accomplish this. If my theory is correct, this is an unreasonable goal because we are not likely to succeed. The decision to do this is, in part, a reflection of the American society in which the spirit of egalitarianism has been taken too far. The notion that "all men are created equal" is patently absurd. All men are *not* created equal. Not only are there differences in height, weight, eye color, and hair color, but there are formidable differences in cognitive capacity. I am certainly in agreement that all men (and women) should be *treated* as equal before the law regarding the administration of justice; but this is quite different from the notion of all men being *created* equal. Another factor that has contributed to the this unfortunate situation is the upward mobility of our American society and the view that every person should be given every opportunity to reach his or her highest potential. Although I have no criticism of a society that provides *opportunities* for the fullfilment of such aspirations, I believe that proper recognition is not being given to the reality that some people will never reach certain goals because they are neurologically and physically incapable of doing so. It is well to recognize such inferiority and not deny it.

Another reason why there are more children being diagnosed GMBDS in the United States than in other countries relates to our educational system. In many countries there is a greater acceptance of the reality that not all children should be given a higher education, because of the appreciation that not all children are intellectually capable of profiting from such education. In many countries, somewhere between the ages of 9 and 11, children are often divided into 3 educational tracks. The most demanding track is for those who will continue with an intense academically oriented program in preparation for ultimate attendance at a college or university. The least rigorous track is for those children who have shown little or no competence or ability for formal academics. They are therefore given a few more years of 3R education and then channeled for training in trades or careers that are much less academically demanding. And the middle category falls somewhere in between. Although there is a possibility of "switching tracks" it is not very common.

Although one could argue that the system may result in potential geniuses being lost, one could argue also that it serves the greatest good for the greatest number. Whatever the advantages and disadvantages of the system, it certainly has the advantage of recognizing at the outset the reality of the existence and importance of the bell-shaped curves I have emphasized so much previously. One of this system's main advantages is that it protects children from the ego-debasing experiences of being considered to have a disease when, in fact, they do not. Children in the US who are diagnosed GMBDS are not labeled as such (or its equivalent) in most other countries. They are put in the 3rd track, which is generally a far more acceptable position. They are not subjected to taunts such as "retard" or "ment" and they are not exposed to the mortifying experience of being surrounded by others with whom they will invariably compare themselves unfavorably. They do not have to dread daily attendance at a school where they are ever anticipating public humiliation from teachers who will inevitably be asking them to perform at levels beyond their innate capacities. Although it may sound like a very undemocratic thing to say, I believe that we would do well to institute this system in the United States.

My theory has profound implications for psychiatry as well. Many psychiatrists prescribe psychostimulant medication for the treatment of some of the primary neurologically based symptoms such as hyperactivity and attentional impairment. Their belief and hope (misguided, I believe) is that reduction of these symptoms will also somehow improve learning. This has never been conclusively established and never will, I believe, because the primary learning deficits are genetically based and these medications do not, I believe, affect the genes. Perhaps some day we will be able to do this. This is not to deny that the child who is less active may learn more. It is to deny that psychostimulant medication directly improves visual processing, auditory processing, and reasoning capacity. Some believe that doing treatment of these primary symptoms will obviate the development of the secondary psychogenic symptoms. Others recognize that this is not the case and attempt to treat these secondary symptoms psychotherapeutically. This examiner is in the latter category (R.A. Gardner, 1973a, 1973b, 1974a, 1974b, 1975a, 1975b, 1975c and 1986). Furthermore, I presently have in preparation a book devoted to this form of treatment, *Psychotherapy of the Psychogenic Problems of Children with Neurologically Based Learning Disabilities*. However, we could contribute significantly to the prevention of the secondary psychogenic disorders from arising in the first place if the aforementioned 3-track educational system were utilized. Accordingly, I strongly recommend that therapists do whatever they can to modify our educational system. This would be a good example of "preventive psychiatry." Otherwise, we will just continue to "pick up the pieces" and attempt to treat the unnecessary sequelae of an iatrogenic disorder that need not have existed in the first place. It is a disorder artificially created by denial of reality by educators and other professionals. This book is an offering in the service of such modification of our educational program. It can be viewed then as a volume on preventive psychiatry.

Another factor in American society that has contributed to the grief of GMBDS children is the widespread worship of the so-called "college education." Many families believe that all their children should go to college and that child who does not do so brings disgrace to the family. This attitude is also based on a denial of reality. However, there are hundreds of colleges that cater to this demand. Where there is a customer who is willing to pay money for something, there will always be someone who will be willing to provide the service and charge handsomely for it. There are colleges for LD children and there are even colleges for retarded children. As long as these institutions exist "at the end of the road" there will be a perpetuation of the attempts to bring GMBDS children up to levels beyond their capability.

I believe that most colleges in the United States are not serving primarily as educational institutions; rather, they are serving as what I call "winter camps" for immature youngsters. Most youngsters who are attending college are not going to be educated; but are sent there for another four years of prolongation of their dependent state. We have a unique disease in the United States which I call *the college disease*. Millions of parents believe that it is crucial that their children attend college and actually believe that the schools to which they are sending their children are actually serving educational purposes. As mentioned, when there is a demand for something, there will always be individuals who will be pleased to provide a supply of the product, especially when there is good money to be made in the business. Most collegiate institutions in the United States are basically businesses. Yet, they have their academic hierarchy: there are assistant professors, associate professors, and full professors. They have their college-style buildings (especially red brick and ivy), their alumni associations, their football teams, and their fund-raising campaigns. But the vast majority of students are not there to learn; rather, they are there primarily to have a "good time"—which often includes significant indulgence in alcohol, drugs, and sex. When they are not engaged in these activities, they go through the motions of attending classes, but little is learned. Grade inflation insures that even those with borderline intelligence will get high grades, and it is rare for someone to flunk out. And why should they fail? Does one kick a good customer out of the store? If a customer's parents are willing to continue to pay for the services provided, it would be self-destructive on the college's part to cut off a predictable supply of money because of a student's "failure" to consume the product being offered.

It is important for the reader to appreciate the use of the word *most*. I did not say that *all* collegiate institutions are in the summer camp category. If I had to give a percentage of those academic institutions in the United States that fit the above description, I would say that it is in the 75 to 80 percent range. Furthermore, the supply of such institutions presently is greater than the demand. Accordingly, all but the most prestigious institutions are scrounging around looking for customers. All the youngster need do is sign up for the SATs and he or she will soon find the mailbox filled with solicitations from colleges. Most often, the youngster's scores (no matter how low) are not a determinant of whether or not he or she will be placed on the institution's mailing list. In fact, for many, the lower the scores the happier the institution because it recognizes that it will have a better shot at attracting the inferior student than the one who has proven him- or herself genuinely worthy of a bona fide collegiate experience.

In this highly competitive market GMBDS children are highly sought after. There are institutions in which the concept of the neurologically based learning disability was practically unknown a few years ago. However, there suddenly appeared a "program" for these youngsters, often taught by people who had little if any training in this area. The diplomas that the GMBDS children ultimately receive from these institutions is most often of little commercial value with regard to its providing them with a greater opportunity for a job. Although the youngster and the parents may derive some ostensible comfort and pride from the knowledge that the child is now a "college graduate," inwardly they know that the document is worthless and this cannot but be ego-debasing to such youngsters because they know in their hearts how meaningless is the document their parents have bought for them. Parents who are judicious enough to protect themselves from affliction with the college disease remove their youngsters from a highly demanding academic college-oriented track in early adolescence and make every attempt to place the child in a trade or skill-oriented program with only minimal emphasis on further formal academic training. They thereby help the youngster prepare for functioning in a real world, as a self-sufficient human being who is more likely to gain a sense of pride in his or her accomplishments.

The theory has formidable implications for the therapist. As long as one views ADD children to have a basic neurophysiological defect, one is likely to assume that psychotherapy is not indicated as a primary treatment and consider only psychostimulant medication. If, however, one considers valid the theory proposed here then one may view these children's attentional deficit to be primarily related to the fact that their genetic programming is such that sitting 6 to 7 hours a day is an unnatural constraint. In addition, one will then be more likely to consider psychogenic factors to be operative. When investigation reveals that this is also the case, then psychotherapy will be warranted. In some cases such inquiry may lead the examiner to conclude that the genetic programming factor need not be invoked at all because the attentional impairment can reasonably be explained as related to psychogenically induced tensions and anxieties. And this is an extremely important point. Many, if not most, of the children diagnosed as having ADD have psychogenic problems and are not receiving psychotherapy, but merely psychostimulant medication. This is a cop-out. It is a seemingly easy solution to a complex problem. It is a manifestation of a trend in recent years in psychiatry to view psychiatric disorders as organic and avoid thereby the more time-consuming and expensive course of detailed inquiry and psychotherapeutic intervention.

THREE

Assessing Objectively the Effects of Psychostimulant Medication on Selective Symptoms of the Group of Mimimal Brain Dysfunction Syndromes

The remaining 2 chapters of this book will be devoted to studies of mine that provide objective data that lend support to some of the ideas presented in my theory. Obviously, 2 chapters in 1 book would not suffice to prove the whole theory; hundreds of investigators working throughout their lives would probably be necessary to accomplish that. My purpose here, then, is to provide some data that lend support to my views on the alleged attention-sustaining impairment of these children. Although Figure 2-1 suggests that I am focusing on a relatively small aspect of their problems, the ADD diagnosis has enjoyed widespread enthusiasm, so much so that it may be the most commonly diagnosed disorder of children in the

1980s. If it is indeed a myth that the disorder exists (as my theory suggests) then focus on this relatively small entity has important implications. The main data that lend support to my conclusion that ADD as an *isolated disease entity* is rare or non-existent was derived from data that led me to this conclusion. The data was derived from studies which were set up with the assumption that ADD does indeed exist and that its diagnosis and treatment should be more objective. More specifically, these studies were embarked upon in order to find instruments that would be useful in monitoring objectively the psychostimulant medication that is considered to help children sustain attention. In this chapter I will describe in detail the basic format of the study and in Chapter Four I will discuss my findings, especially with regard to their implications for my theory. Again, the findings about ADD came first and their application to my theory came second.

In the late 1960s and 1970s a number of questionnaires were developed to ascertain objectively children's activity levels. In 1980, with the publication of DSM-III, these same questionnaires were utilized to diagnose ADD in that hyperactivity and ADD came to be viewed by many examiners as manifestations of the same deficiency. DSM-III suggests that the 2 may not necessarily coexist in that one can diagnose ADD with *or* without hyperactivity. However, the fundamental disease process is considered to be ADD and most examiners soon came to the conclusion that there was no such disease entity as ADD without hyperactivity. In practice, then, the notion that ADD and hyperactivity were one and the same gave support and sanction to those who would use the previously developed hyperactivity scales for the assessment of ADD. The Conners' scales, to be described below, are the best known examples of this phenomenon. The same questionnaires that were used in the 70s to assess for the presence of hyperactivity were immediately utilized in the 80s for the assessment of ADD and are still being utilized for this purpose. The most well-known scales are The Werry-Weiss-Peters Activity Scale (J.S. Werry, 1968); The Bell, Waldrop, and Weller Rating System (R.Q. Bell et al., 1972); The Conners' Teacher Rating Scale (C.K. Conners, 1969); The Conners' Parent Questionnaire (C.K. Conners, 1973); and Davids' Rating Scale for Hyperkinesis (A. Davids, 1971). I have serious reservations about these scales and have not personally found them useful.

One objection relates to rater reliability. When filling out such a scale the rater is often placed in the position of making almost impossible discriminations. He or she may be asked questions about whether a child's behavior falls into the category "just a little" as opposed to the category "pretty much" (Conners' Teacher Rating Scale and Conners' Parent Questionnaire). All 6 items of the Davids' scale (1971) ask the rater to differentiate "slightly less" from "less" and "much less." Especially on scales that have many items (The Conners' Parent Questionnaire has 94), the rater is going to fatigue and become less thoughtful regarding the answers. I would go further and state that if, immediately after completing one of these scales, a parent or teacher were asked to repeat his or her answers on a new blank form, there would be significant differences in the responses, especially on the longer scales.

A number of years ago I conducted a study (R.A. Gardner, 1969) in which parents were asked to write their answers to 28 true-false questions. Immediately after the test was completed I verbally reviewed each question with the parent. I found that 10-15% of the responses had to be changed. Either the parent did not understand the question and yet marked an answer so as not to reveal his or her ignorance, or the question was understood but the parent placed an answer in the box inappropriate to the intended response. This was a simple true-false questionnaire, involving only a choice between 2 responses. The errors introduced into a scale that allows for 4 possible responses must be greater. R.M. Simpson (1944) found significant differences among raters when applying the category "frequently." Twenty-five percent of raters used the term to denote events occurring *up to* 40% of the time and another 25% used it to refer only to events occuring *over* 80% of the time. This so-called objective data is then fed into computers and serves as the basis for some of the most sophisticated statistical analyses. The conclusions derived from such studies must be suspect considering the questionable value of the data on which they are primarily based.

Subjective elements are introduced in other ways. The raters' own background and experience must contribute to whether he or she will consider many behavioral items unusual or excessive. People from European and Asian backgrounds consider most American children to be excessively active, and they consider permissiveness of American parents to be the cause. D.F. Klein and R. Gittelman-Klein (1974) found that mothers tended to deny manifestations of hyperactivity when filling out such scales and gave their children lower scores than social workers. And most examiners agree that teachers are likely to see behavior as more severe when it causes trouble or conflict. By what criteria does one decide whether a child "talks excessively" (Werry-Weiss-Peters Activity Scale)? Where does the normal frequency end and the pathological begin for such behavior as "restlessness during church/movies," "restlessness during shopping," and "disrupt's other's play" (Werry-Weiss-Peters Activity Scale)?

My most important objection, however, relates to the basic validity of these scales — whether or not they actually measure hyperactivity. Some of the items are clearly related to hyperactive behavior, such as questions about wiggling, getting up and down from the seat, interrupting, and fidgeting. However, finding the point where the normal degree of such behavior ends and the pathological begins is often very difficult, if not impossible. More importantly, it is the inclusion of items that have little or nothing to do with hyper-

activity or minimal brain dysfunction that lessens significantly the value of such scales for diagnostic purposes, as well
as for determining treatment progress. The Bell, Waldrop,
and Weller Rating System includes "emotional aggression"
and "nomadic play" as 2 of the 7 items in their hyperactivity
scale. Although both of these *may* be seen in children with
GMBDS, they are certainly seen with significant frequency in
children with purely psychogenic problems. The Conners'
Parent Questionnaire, which is purported to have diagnosed
hyperactivity in 74% of 133 cases (C.K. Conners, 1970), has
such items as headaches, stomachaches, vomiting, loose
bowels, bullying, plays with sex organs, truancy, stealing,
firesetting, pouts and sulks, perfectionism, shy, mean, and
daydreams. These, and many of the other symptoms listed on
the Conners' scale, are primarily, if not entirely, psychogenic
in etiology. Although it may be true that GMBDS children,
because of their basic handicap, are more likely to have such
superimposed psychogenic problems than normals, does not
justify including such items in a scale designed to be used
with children with this disorder. The tendency on the part of
the rater has been to assume that these symptoms are an intrinsic part of GMBDS and not differentiate between those
symptoms that are primary manifestations and those that are
secondary psychogenic. Conners' scale mixes them all
together.

C.K. Conners (1969) has factor analyzed the 39 items on
his Teacher Rating Scale (which includes such items as self-
ish, daydreams, "tattles," steals, lies, appears to lack leader-
ship, and shy) and has delineated five clusters: I, aggressive
conduct; II, daydreaming-inattentive; III, anxious-fearful; IV,
hyperactivity; and V, sociable-cooperative. The factor IV
group not only includes items that are traditionally associated
with hyperactivity (sits diddling with small objects, hums and
makes other odd noises, restless, and overactive) but others
that I do not consider to be intrinsic to neurological impair-

ment (disturbs other children, teases other chidren and interferes with their activities, excessive demands for teacher's
attention, submissive, and overly anxious to please.) Again, it
is probably true that GMBDS children are more likely than
normals to have these symptoms. However, as discussed in
Chapter One, the clear distinction between primary organic
manifestations and secondary psychological problems is very
important for etiological understanding as well as for therapeutic purposes. Scales that clump them together easily lead
the user of the scale to forget about making this important
differentiation.

Saxon et al. (1976) studied the construct validity of three
of the aforementioned rating scales (C.K. Conners, 1969; A.
Davids, 1971; R.Q. Bell et al., 1972) by determining if there
were any correlations between parents' ratings on the scales
and 2 more objective laboratory measures of hyperactivity.
Laboratory measurements of hyperactivity were determined
by 1) actometers (self-winding calendar watches that had
been converted to motion recorders), and 2) ultrasonic motion
detectors (burglar alarm systems that quantitatively measured the amount of the child's movement in a 9 ft × 11 ft.
room). They found no significant correlation between the
child's activity as measured by either of the 2 devices and activity level as determined by the parents' using any of the 3
scales. It is of interest that Saxon et al. used the total Conners
Teachers' Rating Scale, not just the factor IV items, thus confirming my previously expressed belief that the more common use of the Conners' scale is to view all the items as being
in some way correlated with hyperactivity. D. Ross and
S. Ross (1976) share my views regarding the limitation of
these 4 scales and provide an excellent discussion of their
deficiencies.

In spite of their obvious drawbacks, these scales (especially the Conners' scales) presently enjoy great popularity
among researchers. They are frequently used in research on

the efficacy of psychostimulant medication and often serve as the primary criterion for evaluating the potency of such drugs. Therefore, the value of a drug to reduce hyperactivity is being tested by scales that have not been well demonstrated to measure hyperactivity. Accordingly, the conclusions that are being reached by such studies are of dubious value. In short, I consider these scales to be of doubtful validity and questionable reliability.

THE PSYCHOSTIMULANT MEDICATION ASSESSMENT BATTERY

Introductory Comments

Since the 1950s the hyperactivity label has been very much in vogue. In the 1970s I developed my Steadiness Tester in order to assess objectively for the presence of this symptom. Although the instrument proved useful for this purpose, it proved more useful for the objective monitoring of the effects of psychostimulant medication on hyperactivity (R.A. Gardner, et al., 1979). Unfortunately, the Steadiness Tester has never enjoyed widespread utilization for this purpose, mainly I believe because of its high price ($280). In the early 1980s, immediately after the publication of DSM-III, the ADD diagnosis quickly became epidemic. Because of the high price of the Steadiness Tester, I began to look for less expensive instruments – especially pencil and paper – that could be used to monitor objectively the affects of psychostimulant medication on ADD. However, I realized that before I could utilize an instrument for such monitoring I would first have to ascertain whether a particular pencil and paper test was indeed sensitive to psychostimulant medication and, if so, if it could then be used to monitor such medication. It was with these purposes in mind that I developed *The Psychostimulant Medication Assessment Battery* (PMAB).

The General Purposes of the Psychostimulant Medication Assessment Battery

The tests in the *Psychostimulant Medication Assessment Battery (PMAB)* were devised and selected in the hope that they would serve 2 functions. First, 1 or more would prove sensitive to psychostimulant medication, i.e., psychostimulant medication would improve a child's scores, especially if initially deficient. Second, if an instrument did prove sensitive, i.e., if scores could be improved by psychostimulant medication, then an attempt would be made to ascertain whether the instrument could be used to monitor the dosage levels of psychostimulant medication. The hope was that the instrument would be so sensitive to the drug that there would be a direct correlation between the administration of the medication and the child's improvement on the instrument.

The 10 instruments in the PMAB were selected because they had been reported in the literature to assess functions that were improved by psychostimulant medication, namely, hyperactivity, attention deficit, visual perception, and fine motor coordination. There are many instruments that assess these functions. The ones selected for the PMAB were those that lent themselves most readily to use in the office or clinic setting. If the study were to prove successful, then a group of assessment instruments would have been found that are particularly sensitive to detecting the presence of certain "target" symptoms present in GMBDS. The examiner would then be in a position to make statements such as: "Drug X proved useful in improving symptom Y as evidenced by the child's significant improvement on task Z" e.g., "Methylphenidate proved useful in improving Robert's auditory attention, short-term auditory memory, and auditory sequential memory as evidenced by his significant improvement on the Digits Forward section of the Digit Span subtest of the WISC-R (p < .01)." The next step then would be to determine whether the instrument could be useful in monitoring medication, i.e., to ascertain whether even further improvement might be found with higher (or at least different) dosage levels of the medication.

The Areas of Deficit Assessed by the Psychostimulant Medication Assessment Battery

Attentional impairment is considered by many examiners to be a central problem for children with GMBDS. Parents will often complain that their GMBDS children do not "pay attention." And the efficacy of psychostimulant medication is often attributed to its capacity to help children sustain attention. All tests in the battery rely heavily on concentration capacity. To the best of my knowledge, we do not know whether attentional impairments are generalized and affect all sensory modalities or whether there are specific concentration deficits for each of the sensory modalities, i.e., visual concentration deficit, auditory concentration deficit, etc. The tests in the PMAB may ultimately prove useful in answering this question. Accordingly, 4 tests (#1-#4) assess primarily (but not exclusively) auditory concentration and 3 tests (#4-#6) assess primarily visual concentration.

GMBDS children often exhibit reversals of letters and numbers. A high reversals frequency is seen in children with neurologically based reading disabilities – sometimes referred to as *dyslexia*. Test #7 assesses reversals frequency.

Organizational impairment is a common complaint made by parents and teachers of GMBDS children. They are commonly described as disorganized, confused, lacking follow-through, and always in need of individual attention and structure. Test #8 is included in the battery to assess this function.

Coordination problems are common among GMBDS children. In the classroom visual-motor coordination problems cause these children significant difficulty. Handwriting is poor. Written material is not confined to the lines on the paper. Multiplication and long division is impaired because the child has trouble keeping numbers within proper columns. The deficiency in mechanical skills causes difficulty in art, shop, and cooking classes. On the playing field, as well, visual-motor coordination problesm result in significant humiliation and alienation for the GMBDS child. To ascertain whether psychostimulant medication has an affect on visual-motor coordination, test #9 is included in the battery to assess this function. Some of the aforementioned difficulties are the result of *dyspraxia*—a problem related to the inability of the brain to properly monitor motor function. Test #10 assesses this function.

Parents will often state that the child on psychostimulant medication is more cooperative and "listens to what I say." When parents use the word "listens" in this context, they are generally referring to the child's cooperation rather than to auditory concentration. In order to assess the child's receptivity to following directions, test #2 has been included. however, an auditory concentration factor is also assessed in this test in that it would be difficult, if not impossible, to remove this element from any test that attempts to assess compliance with verbal requests.

Hyperactivity is one of the most commonly described signs of GMBDS. Some believe that hyperactivity is a manifestation of an attentional deficit, i.e., of the child's inability to remain fixed for long on a particular stimulus. The theory holds that psychostimulant medication reducees hyperactivity by improving the child's capacity to sustain attention. Concentrating longer of fewer stimuli, the child does not flit from goal to goal—reducing thereby the activity level. Hyperactivity may also be a neurological manifestation, independent of the attentional factor. Although these 2 causes of hyperactivity may be neurological, psychogenic factors probably contribute in most patients. High activity level is a con-comitant of tension and anxiety. And GMBDS children have much to be fearful about—considering their many impair-ments and the alienation they fear in association with the ex-posure of their deficits. Whatever its etiology, psycho-stimulant medication often reduces hyperactivity. Test #5 utilizes the Steadiness Tester (R.A. Gardner, 1979; R.A. Gardner et al., 1979) to ascertain whether hyperactivity is present and to assess the efficacy of psychostimulant medica-tion in reducing hyperactivity. This instrument will be de-scribed in greater detail later in this chapter.

Ascertaining the Optimum Dosage
Level of Psychostimulant
Medication

Once a decision has been made that the child warrants a trial on medication, then he or she can be considered a candidate for the administration of the PMAB. However, before admin-istering the PMAB subtests, some indication of the child's op-timum dose level of psychostimulant medication should be obtained. This should first be done clinically. On a weekend, when the parents have the greatest opportunity to observe the child, a relatively low dose should be administered in the morning. For example, on Saturday morning 5 mg. of methyl-phenidate might be administered. The parents should be ad-vised to observe for a number of possible reactions. If the dose is too high, the child might exhibit agitation, headache, palpi-tations, or generalized irritability. Occasionally, psychomotor retardation ("He's like a zombie") is seen if the dose is too high. If the dose is too low, no changes will be observed. If the dose is adequate, there may be a reduction in activity level, improved concentration, reduced impulsivity, increased re-ceptivity to attending to what the parents say, and greater compliance with their requests. What happens on Saturday will determine what dose they give on Sunday. If 5 mg. on Saturday produced manifestations of excessive dosage (unusual at the 5 mg. level) then a smaller dose, such as 2½ mg., should be administered. If there was no observable change, then 7½ or 10 mg. of methylphenidate might still be tried on Sunday in order to determine whether one can get even greater improvement. Of course, still higher doses might be necessary before clinical improvement is observed. It may take 3 or 4 days of clinical testing before one obtains an optimum dose.

Ascertaining the Period of Optimum Efficacy of Psychostimulant Medication

If the examiner does not have a Steadiness Tester available, then the dose level obtained by the aforementioned clinical method should be used and testing should be given at that time interval which clinically appeared to have been optimum (usually between 1 and 3 hours). However, a more objective assessment of optimum dosage and period of optimum efficacy can be accomplished by utilizing such instruments as this examiner's Steadiness Tester. A baseline of 2-to-3 scores is obtained to confirm that the child's score is indeed elevated. The well-rested child will generally provide a baseline whose points do not differ by more than 20% from one another. There are children, however, who exhibit wider variability of response. For such children a few more trials may be necessary to establish a meaningful baseline range. If, however, the child's score is not elevated then this instrument cannot be used to assess drug dosage level. This does not mean that psychostimulant medication cannot be useful for the child; it only means that the child does not exhibit one of the symptoms (hyperactivity/attentional deficit) for which psychostimulant medication can be useful. The child may still benefit from the medication in other areas of dysfunction—such as compliance and impulsivity.

If the child's score is elevated (the usual case for GMBDS children), and consistently so, then the Steadiness Tester can be utilized to determine the optimum dose. First, the *clinically determined* optimum dose of medication is administered (usually 5 mg. of dextroamphetamine sulfate or 10 mg. of methylphenidate). The drug should be given early in the morning in order to approximate as closely as possible the school situation. It is also preferable that a score be obtained just prior to the administration of the drug in order to confirm the reliability of the elevated baseline. Then scores are obtained after 1 hour, 2 hours, 3 hours, 4 hours, and (if necessary) 5 hours. Generally, a curve is obtained (Figure 3-1) that will provide the examiner with information about drug efficacy. If the dip is formidable, especially if down to the normal range, one can conclude that the child is a good responder. The time it takes to achieve optimum improvement can also be determined from the curve. Generally, the greatest improvement occurs between 1 and 3 hours, but it may vary. If there is no particular change, one way or the other, then the dose has probably not been high enough and the test should be readministered on another day with a higher dose. If the performance deteriorates, i.e., the child's scores get higher, then the guessed dose has probably been too high (causing agitation) and the test should be administered on another day with a lower dose. (This is rare if one starts with 5 mg. of dextroamphetamine sulfate or 10 mg. of methylphenidate.) The 1- to 2-hour post-medication testing period suggested for the PMAB is based on the usual period of optimum improvement based on Steadiness Tester performance. However, if the examiner has good reason to believe that a different time lag should be utilized (either from clinical experience or objective testing) then that lag should be used. If the testing series has to be repeated because the initial dose did not prove optimal, it is most often not necessary to repeat every step. For example, the parent can be instructed to administer the medication at home and then to bring the child for the 1-, 2-,

Figure 3-1

RESPONSE TO PSYCHOSTIMULANT MEDICATION AS MEASURED BY THE STEADINESS TESTER
10-year-old boy – 40.3 sec

$\bar{X}_N = 8.80 \pm 7.33$ $+4.3$ S.D. $\ll 10\%$ile (20.17sec)

$\bar{X}_{MBD} = 18.30 \pm 17.45$ $+1.26$ S.D. $\sim 15\%$ile

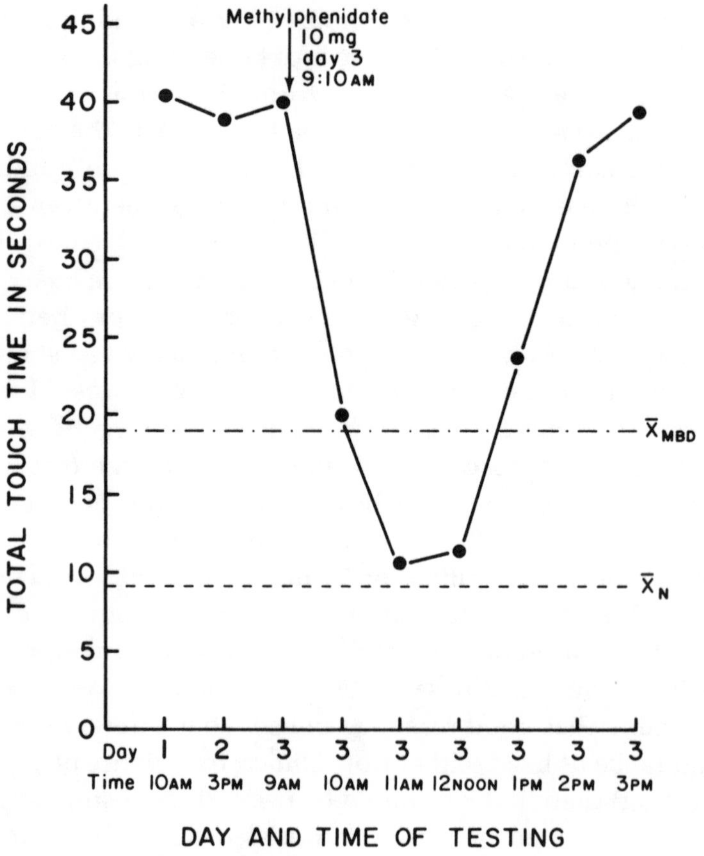

DAY AND TIME OF TESTING

and 3-hour post-medication testings—requiring then only 2 hours of office testing time.

It is important for the examiner to appreciate that assessment for the period of optimum dose efficacy may be complicated by the fact that absorption of psychostimulant medication may be erratic—blood levels and clinical response differing from day to day even after the drug has been administered under seemingly identical conditions. This complication notwithstanding, the examiner does well to try to assess—by combining clinical observations and objective testing—what the optimum dose should be and the time range over which there is maximum drug response.

Minimizing the Practice Effect

Any study that utilizes an instrument for assessing drug efficacy must consider the potential contamination of practice in any improvement observed. To minimize this factor, each test is first administered 3 times before initiating the drug-free and post-drug trials. In order to minimize even further the practice effect 2 additional equivalent (but not identical) forms of 6 of the tests have been prepared. These modified forms are alternated with the standard renditions in the drug assessment phase of the study. Four of the tests do not allow for such variation. Table 3-1 is used to record the child's scores on each of the practice tests. It is hoped that the 3 trials will be sufficient to bring the improvement curve to an asymptote, so that further improvement under drug conditions will be primarily (if not exclusively) a manifestation of drug effect.

Assessment for the Presence of Impairment

In order to determine whether an impairment is present on any of the 10 tests, the examiner should record the normal

Table 3-1 Psychostimulant Medication Assessment Battery Tabulation of Data

Assessment Instrument	Norm.	Score	Defic.	Practice Trials	Drug free 1	Post drug 2	Drug free 3	Post drug 4	Drug free 5	Post drug 6	p
1. Word Span		A		A	A	C	B	A	C	B	
2. Compliance with Serial Verbal Instructions		A		A	A	C	B	A	C	B	
3. Digit Span Digits Forward (WISC-R)		A		A	A	C	B	A	C	B	
4. Digit Span Digits Backward (WISC-R)		A		A	A	C	B	A	C	B	
5. Steadiness Tester		A		A	A	A	A	A	A	A	
6. Cancellation of Rapidly Recurring Target Figures		A		A	A	C	B	A	C	B	
7. Reversals Frequency Test, Recognition		A		A	A	A	A	A	A	A	
8. Block Design (WISC-R)		A		A	A	C	B	A	C	B	
9. Purdue Pegboard		A		A	A	A	A	A	A	A	
10. Development Test of Visual-Motor Integration		A		A	A	A	A	A	A	A	

Name ___ Age ___ years ___ months Sex ___ Drug ___ Dose ___ score for the child's age in the *Norm.* column of Table 3-1 and compare it with the child's original assessment score, which should be recorded in the *Score* column. An impairment is considered present if the child's score is below the 20th percentile, and/or more than 1 s.d. below the mean, and/or 2 or more years below grade level, and/or at an age-equivalent below 80% of the child's chronological age. If *any* of the above criteria are satisfied, then a *Yes* (or Y) is recorded in the *Defic.* column. If no deficiency is present, then a *No* (or N) is recorded. And if the results are equivocal, then a ± should be entered.

At this point the examiner must decide which of the 10 areas of deficit warrant further study. If the deficiency is severe and/or other instruments in the examiner's battery support the conclusion that a deficit is present in the particular area, then further assessment is strongly indicated.

Administration of the Practice Trials

When a decision has been made that further study is warranted, then 2 more trials should be administered. This should be accomplished with 2 more administrations of the original Form A format. This is done to keep the Forms B and C modifications "pure" for the subsequent drug assessment trials. If, for research purposes, the examiner has chosen to assess the child's performance in nondeficient areas, then the Form A administration should be repeated twice more as well. If the number of deficiency areas is low, then the examiner is likely to have more time available for conducting the study of nondeficient areas. Confining the study to deficient areas is of immediate value to the child in that it can provide information about whether psychostimulant medication is helping that particular child in the areas of deficiency. Assessing drug effect in areas of nondeficiency should prove useful for the purposes of a broader research program in which the data might ultimately be utilized, e.g., studies assessing the effects of drugs on normal scores. In both cases the repetitions of practice trials should be done on separate days to maintain consistency with the drug trial phase wherein such time separations are crucial. The patient's scores on the practice repetitions are recorded in the Practice Trials 2 and 3 columns of Table 3-1.

If repeated administration of the test results in a deficient score being brought into the normal range (not uncommon), the examiner should not automatically conclude that the deficiency is not present. It must be remembered that the original instrument was standardized on a population in which the test was administered on 1 occasion only. The score in such administration does not represent the 2nd or the 3rd trial. If the child's original score was in the borderline range ($\pm$) or the examiner has reason to believe that a bona fide impairment exists, then the child's scores on other instruments must be studied in order to ascertain whether an impairment genuinely exists in the particular area. In such circumstances that particular PMAB test cannot be used for psychostimulant medication assessment.

Administering the Tests Under Drug-Free and Post-Drug Conditions

The drug-free and post-drug trials should be administered on separate days (preferably spaced by 2 or 3 days) to insure that the child is no longer under the influence of medication when tested in the drug-free state. The PMAB's reliability can be assessed only by repeating the drug-free/post-drug sequence twice more. This appears to be the minimum number of repetitions necessary to provide meaningful statistical analysis of the data. Such repetition is also important because of the possible presence of residual practice effect—the 3 aforementioned trials notwithstanding. Repetition is also warranted because of the erratic way in which psychostimulant medication is absorbed from the gastrointestinal track—blood levels differing from day to day even after identical doses are given under seemingly identical conditions. Depending upon the age of the child and his or her speed of execution of the tasks, the 10 tests can generally be administered between 60 and 90 minutes. Of course, if fewer tests are administered, the time would be shorter. Because children are likely to be less alert the later in the day they are tested, it is preferable to test the child in the morning. If this is difficult to achieve, then the tests should be administered at approximately the same time of the day on each occasion.

As mentioned, 3 variations have been prepared for 6 of the tests (#1, #2, #3, #4, #6, and #8), whereas variations were not feasible for 4 of the tests (#5, #7, #9, and #10). Each of the 3 forms has been designated A, B, and C. The A form is the one that has been initially standardized. The B and C forms are the variations devised by this examiner. Careful study of the variation forms (see section in which the 10 tests are described) will reveal that the differences between the modifications and the original have been created to minimize practice effect, but in no way alter content. During the initial phase, in which the originally standardized test is repeated twice more to minimize practice effect, only the original rendition (Form A) should be administered. Of course, if the examiner has chosen not to assess drug effect on tests which are in the normal range, then these tests need not be repeated. When drug effect is assessed (in both deficit and nondeficit areas) then the alternative renditions (Forms B and C) are administered.

In order to minimize further the practice effect, a special sequencing of the 3 forms should be administered over the 6 trials involving drug-free and post-drug assessments. The following sequence should be followed:

> Trial 1 - Drug-free Form A
> Trial 2 - Post-drug Form C
> Trial 3 - Drug-free Form B
> Trial 4 - Post-drug Form A
> Trial 5 - Drug-free Form C
> Trial 6 - Post-drug Form B

Using this design, each of the forms A, B, and C is administered in a drug-free state and each is administered in the post-drug state as well. When a statistical analysis is performed on such data, neither the drug-free nor the post-drug category is overly represented by variations of the instrument that might be biased in a particular direction. Accordingly, it is extremely important that the examiner adhere strictly to the aforementioned sequence of administration.

After the series has been repeated 6 times (3 drug-free trials alternating with 3 post-drug trials), one ascertains whether the drug has produced significant improvement. Ideally, these 6 trials should be done on 6 separate days. And, as mentioned, it is preferable that there be a 2-3 day hiatus between the days on which drugs have been given and the days of the drug-free trials. However, under special circumstances, when time and distance make such multiple trips difficult, the examiner might perform the drug-free trial in the early part of the day, administer the drug at the end of the testing period, and then retest after that interval which the Steadiness Tester has revealed to be the optimum time for testing under drug conditions. Although this procedure adds the complication of testing taking place at different times of the day, I suspect that it will not seriously compromise the evaluation.

Ascertaining Statistically the
Significance of the Results

A t-test with correlated samples is used and the probability that changes for a particular subject are significant is recorded in the p column of Table 3-1. If a computer is not available then the Sandler's A-statistic may be utilized. Sandler's formula for assessing t-test with correlated samples:

$$A = \frac{\Sigma\,D^2}{(\Sigma\,D)^2}$$

D is the difference between the drug-free and the post-drug scores for each of the 3 comparisons. Referring to Sandler's table of levels of significance for two-tailed test ($N-1 = 2$), A is significant at a given level if it is *equal to* or *less than* the following values:

A	p
0.412	.10
0.369	.05
0.347	.02
0.340	.01
0.334	.001

Calculated p values are recorded in the extreme right column of Table 3-1. The table below tabulates a typical calculation:

Trial	after	before	D	D²
1	23	30	+7	49
2	24	31	+7	49
3	24	30	+6	36
Σ			+20	134

$$\text{Sandler's A} = \frac{\Sigma D^2}{(\Sigma D)^2} = \frac{134}{(20)^2} = \frac{134}{400} = 0.335$$

In the above calculation p < .01 because 0.335 is below 0.340, the Sandler's A figure that corresponds to the .01 level. We can conclude here that the drug did produce a significant change in the child's performance.

Another example:

Trial	after	before	D	D²
1	18	22	+4	16
2	23	21	−2	4
3	27	2	+2	4
Σ			+4	24

$$\text{Sandler's A} = \frac{\Sigma D^2}{(\Sigma D)^2} = \frac{24}{16} = 1.500$$

Because Sandler's A would have to be below 0.412 to reach the p < .10 level, we can conclude here that the drug did not produce significant changes.

The protocol described above is utilized for assessing drug efficacy for an individual child. For research purposes, the same program should be administered with placebos with another child. This would be another way to minimize the practice effect with data that suggests drug efficacy. A statistical comparison between the drug and placebo groups should provide further information about the value of the PMAB in assessing the efficacy of psychostimulant medication.

When the battery is completed, the data in Table 3-1 enable the examiner to ascertain whether psychostimulant medication has been effective in improving a child's score in a particular area of deficit. In addition, if the tests were administered in areas in which there was no impairment, it can enable the examiner to determine whether there has been improvement as well in areas in which there was no deficit. Each child's scores has immediate clinical value with regard to answering the question of whether psychostimulant medication is efficacious for that particular child in improving functioning in specific areas. In addition, statistical analysis of Table 3-1 data for large numbers of children should prove useful with regard to our ability to make some general statements about the efficacy of psychostimulant medication for improving a child's performance in areas of deficiency commonly present in GMBDS children. Furthermore, if ample data have been collected on a large number of children regarding the effect of psychostimulant medication on nondeficient areas, then information on this issue will also emerge from the study.

Equipment Necessary for Administering the Psychostimulant Medication Assessment Battery

In the next section, I will describe in detail the 10 ten tests of the PMAB. An attempt will be made to provide examiners with as much information as possible in order that they themselves will be able to administer the tests. In addition, normative data are provided for all of the instruments with the exception of test #8 (Block Design subtest of the WISC-R) and #10 (The Developmental Test of Visual-Motor Integration). For the latter instruments the normative data are provided by the manufacturers.

It was my initial aim to utilize only pencil-and-paper tests in the PMAB. However, some additional equipment proved to be necessary. Most of the instruments are still in the pencil-and-paper category and can be administered by the examiner from information and normative data provided with each instrument. However, some additional equipment is necessary for the administration of some of the tests. Listed below are the names of these instruments, their catalogue numbers, and the places where they can be obtained.

> Test #5. *The Steadiness Tester* (Cat. No. 32019)
> Lafayette Instrument Co.
> P.O. Box 1279
> Lafayette, Indiana 47902

Test #8. *Weschsler Intelligence Scale for Children-Revised (Block Design)*
The Psychological Corp.
555 Academic Court
San Antonio, Texas 78204

Test #9. *The Purdue Pegboard* (Cat. No. 32020)
Lafayette Instrument Co.
P.O. Box 1279
Lafayette, Indiana 47902

Test #10. *Developmental Test of Visual-Motor Integration (Beery and Buktenica)*
Follett Publishing Co.
100 West Washington Blvd.
Chicago, Illinois 60607

**The Ten Tests in the
Psychostimulant Medication
Assessment Battery**

1. Word Span (Gardner) When administering *The Word Span Test*, the child is presented with progressively longer sequences of 1-syllable words. These words are generally understood by the average 4-year-old child. The child is then asked to repeat as many of the words as possible—immediately after the presentation. The instrument assesses auditory attention, short-term memory, and auditory sequential memory.

The test begins with the examiner providing the child with these instructions (or words to this effect): "This is a test to see how good you are at remembering longer and longer lists of words. Listen carefully to the words I'll be saying and then try to repeat them all as soon as I finish. It's important to try to remember *all* of the words on each list. It's important also to remember the words in the same order as I say them. For example, if I say, 'fish, tooth' and you say, 'tooth, fish' you will have changed the words around, and you won't get credit. You'll get it wrong. You also don't get credit if you forget any of the words on each of the lists. Okay, let's start!"

The test begins with the examiner presenting each of the 3 2-word sequences. The child's scores are recorded on the score sheet (Table 3-2). The examiner then presents the 3 3-word sequences and continues until the child fails to obtain credit for all 3 sequences at a specific level e.g., all 3 5-word se-

Table 3-2   The Word Span Test — Score Sheet

1. Word Span				
Discontinue after failure of all 3 sequences at the same level.				
Level		Points		Subtotal
2	2	2	2	6
				6
3	3	3	3	9
				15
4	4	4	4	12
				27
5	5	5	5	15
				42
6	6	6	6	18
				60
7	7	7	7	21
				81
8	8	8	8	24
				105
9	9	9	9	27
				132

Form A B C

Total
Score

quences. Again, credit is only given if all the words in the sequence are recalled *and* repeated in the correct order. No credit is given if the order is incorrect, even though all the words have been recalled. Scores are tallied on the score sheet (Table 3-2). The normative data (Table 3-3) are used only to ascertain whether or not a child's initial scores are in the normal range. For simplicity, the raw scores only are used for assessing the effects of psychostimulant medication.

Table 3-3   The Word Span Test (Gardner)

	Normative Data — Means and Standard Deviations					
	Boys			Girls		
Age	*N*	*Mean*	*SD*	*N*	*Mean*	*SD*
5-5½	9	19.89	7.80	6	16.50	3.55
5½-6	13	22.15	9.75	10	18.60	5.26
6-6½	18	24.06	8.65	13	23.15	5.45
6½-7	27	27.48	18.01	17	22.76	7.68
7-7½	23	26.39	8.21	17	27.00	8.27
7½-8	25	27.28	9.22	25	32.64	9.42
8-8½	31	28.71	8.98	25	28.72	7.09
8½-9	24	30.21	9.19	23	28.65	7.23
9-9½	24	30.67	10.47	20	30.90	8.55
9½-10	25	33.36	9.42	14	28.21	8.22
10-10½	17	34.88	11.04	21	28.86	10.37
10½-11	22	32.95	6.75	16	32.75	8.14
11-11½	14	32.00	8.53	16	28.38	6.31
11½-12	17	34.53	7.10	8	34.50	5.00
12-12½	9	38.11	8.21	11	37.18	13.09
12½-13	8	34.75	9.00	9	38.33	12.10
13-13½	10	37.70	13.33	6	42.83	15.51
13½-14	5	48.00	9.98	7	46.86	13.95
14-14½	4	45.00	14.71	5	39.20	12.61
14½-15	2	52.00	10.00	3	42.33	18.35
15-15½	5	37.20	3.19	3	65.33	28.89
15½-16	5	54.20	17.09	3	44.00	2.83
16-16½	3	59.67	7.41	2	63.00	26.00

Three renditions of the instructions have been prepared (Forms 1A-1C). They are qualitatively identical in that each of the 3 forms has the same composition regarding word content. They differ only in the sequence of presentation of the words. Furthermore, the randomization is confined to the separate levels, i.e., the words utilized at the 2-word level in Form 1A are the same words as those used at the 2-word level in Forms 1B and 1C. However, in the latter forms they are presented in different sequences.

2. Compliance with Serial Verbal Instructions (Gardner) This is a test of the child's ability to comply with a series of verbal instructions. It assesses the capacity to comply serial verbal commands as well as short-term auditory sequential memory. The child is requested to perform simple body tasks readily accomplished by most children over age 3 or 4. It resembles somewhat the childhood game *Simple Simon*. A typical instruction: "Scratch you head, then touch you knee. Go!"

The test begins with the examiner providing the child with these instructions (or words to this effect): "This is a test to see how good you are at doing things I'm going to ask you to do. First stand here (child is placed in a comfortable position) and place your hands on your hips. After you've done the things I've asked you to do, put your hands back on your hips. Now I can only tell you what to do *one* time and *one time only* — so it's important to listen carefully. Also, you must do the things in the same order as I say them. For example, if I say: 'Rub your eye and *then* scratch your head. Go!' you must rub your eye *first* and *then* you must scratch your head. If you do it the other way around, i.e., if you scratch your head first, you don't get credit. You'll get it wrong. Also, it's very important that you wait until I say, 'Go' before starting."

Three renditions of the instructions have been prepared (Forms 2A-2C). They are qualitatively identical in that each of the 3 forms has the identical composition regarding command

WORD SPAN   Form 1A

2   dog   book

2   pen   house

2   doll   hat

3   desk   cat   grass

3   night   pig   clock

3   sun   car   dress

4   horse   ear   goat   star

4   ink   snake   moon   foot

4   nose   milk   rain   cap

5   rat   eye   mud   fly   cup

5   cow   mat   tree   bird   chair

5   ball   toe   kid   pants   tub

6   sock   salt   mouse   tongue   bug   fork

6   day   fish   shirt   saw   child   bag

6   screw   tooth   hen   song   truck   top

7   ice   frog   coat   key   belt   box   spoon

7   boat   door   lips   knife   ox   tool   watch

7   hole   glove   sand   fire   soap   stone   hand

8   crab   wheel   cloud   dice   knee   bowl   boy   hair

8   shoe   bat   snow   dime   bread   ship   ring   glass

8   plane   shirt   toad   kiss   thumb   plate   lamp   girl

9   arm   leg   pot   bike   phone   nail   roof   bell   toy

9   man   sink   horn   floor   pan   mouth   steak   fan   bed

9   stick   block   dish   lunch   pin   bear   neck   nut   rug

WORD SPAN   **F●rm** 1B

2	hat	book
2	doll	pen
2	house	dog

3	dress	cat	night
3	car	clock	desk
3	grass	pig	sun

4	moon	rain	cap	star
4	milk	goat	nose	ink
4	snake	ear	horse	foot

5	cup	cow	tree	chair	toe
5	fly	rat	bird	ball	pants
5	mat	eye	mud	kid	tub

6	bug	day	shirt	saw	screw	song
6	tongue	fork	sock	child	tooth	truck
6	salt	fish	bug	mouse	hen	top

7	key	boat	lips	spoon	ox	hole	fire
7	belt	frog	box	knife	tool	glove	stone
7	coat	door	ice	watch	sand	soap	hand

8	knee	bat	snow	bread	glass	plane	kiss	plate
8	shoe	bowl	crab	hair	ship	dice	toad	lamp
8	boy	wheel	dime	ring	cloud	shirt	thumb	girl

9	floor	bear	horn	stick	phone	bell	mouth	rug	bed
9	arm	toy	sink	neck	dish	fan	lunch	nut	man
9	nail	block	leg	bike	pan	roof	pin	steak	pot

WORD SPAN   Form 1C

2   pen   house

2   book   doll

2   dog   hat

3   night   car   desk

3   pig   cat   grass

3   sun   clock   dress

4   star   milk   ink   foot

4   ear   moon   nose   snake

4   cap   goat   rain   horse

5   toe   chair   fly   ball   mat

5   cow   bird   cup   pants   mud

5   tree   rat   eye   tub   kid

6   saw   fish   tongue   child   salt   top

6   day   bug   sock   tooth   fork   hen

6   song   screw   shirt   truck   bag   mouse

7   frog   spoon   knife   glove   coat   sand   soap

7   lips   ox   tool   stone   key   ice   hand

7   box   boat   hole   door   watch   fire   belt

8   bread   shoe   hair   plate   ship   toad   boy   shirt

8   crab   bat   knee   dice   girl   plane   ring   thumb

8   snow   bowl   glass   lamp   kiss   dime   cloud   wheel

9   pot   man   block   arm   sink   floor   toy   nail   bed

9   rug   bear   leg   horn   bike   stick   dish   phone   pan

9   bell   fan   roof   mouth   lunch   nut   steak   neck   pin

Compliance with Serial Verbal Instructions Form 2A

Credit

1   Rub your nose. Go!

     Hammer a nail. Go!

     Touch your eyebrow. Go!

2   Touch your nose, then stick out your tongue. Go!

     Kiss your hand, then pull your hair. Go!

     Scratch your head, then tickle your arm. Go!

3   Clap your hand, than tap your head, then bend your elbow. Go!

     Touch the floor, then puff out your cheeks, then tickle your arm. Go!

     Snap your fingers, then touch your knee, then pull your ear. Go!

4   Throw a ball, then kiss your hand, then stick out your tongue, then eat soup. Go!

     Rub your eye, then touch your nose, then hit your knee, then kick a ball. Go!

     Touch the floor, then bend your elbow, then hammer a nail, then stamp your foot. Go!

5   Kiss your hand, then snap your fingers, then tap your head, then touch your eyebrow, then puff out your cheeks. Go!

     Touch your knee, then scratch your head, then throw a ball, then clap your hands, then pull your hair. Go!

     Eat soup, then stamp your foot, then stick out your tongue, then pull your ear, then touch your nose. Go!

6   Rub your eye, the hammer a nail, then hit your knee, then rub your nose, then puff out your cheeks, then snap your fingers. Go!

     Rub your nose, then throw a ball, then touch the floor, then rub your eye, then hit your knee, then kick a ball. Go!

     Stamp your foot, then scratch your head, then rub your nose, then touch your knee, then pull your ear, then eat soup. Go!

Compliance with Serial Verbal Instructions Form 2B

Credit

1   Hammer a nail. Go!

Pull your ear. Go!

Hit your knee. Go!

2   Snap your fingers, then touch your knee. Go!

Tap your head, then puff out your cheeks. Go!

Touch your eyebrow, then scratch your head. Go!

3   Stamp your foor, then eat soup, then put your finger in your bellybutton. Go!

Clap your hands, then throw a ball, then stick your finger in your ear. Go!

Rub your eye, then bend your elbow, then tickle your arm. Go!

4   Stamp your foot, then eat soup, then put your finger in your bellybutton, then touch your knee. Go!

Hit your knee, then touch the floor, then kick a ball, then hammer a nail. Go!

Stick out your tongue, then throw a ball, then kiss your hand, then rub your nose. Go!

5   Bend your elbow, then rub your eye, then hit your knee, then hammer a nail, then clap your hands. Go!

Rub your nose, then kiss your hand, then throw a ball, then stick out your tongue, then kick a ball. Go!

Touch the floor, then eat soup, then pull your ear, then scratch your head, then puff out your cheeks. Go!

6   Snap your fingers, then tickle your arm, then kiss your hand, then rub your nose, then pull your hair, then touch your eyebrow. Go!

Touch your nose, then tap your head, then touch the floor, then puff out your cheeks, then snap your fingers, then stamp your foot. Go!

Scratch your head, then rub your nose, then pull your hair, then touch your knee, then pull your ear, then rub your eye. Go!

Compliance with Serial Verbal Instructions Form 2C

Credit

1　Kiss your hand. Go!

　　Rub your nose. Go!

　　Stamp your foot. Go!

2　Touch the floor, then tap your head. Go!

　　Snap your fingers, then pull your hair. Go!

　　Touch your nose, then touch your eyebrow. Go!

3　Touch your knee, then rub your nose, then kiss your hand. Go!

　　Eat soup, then pull your ear, then scratch your head. Go!

　　Puff out your cheeks, then scratch your head, then throw a ball. Go!

4　Clap your hands, then kick a ball, then stick out your tongue, then pull your hair. Go!

　　Puff out your cheeks, then hammer a nail, then hit your knee, then stamp your foot. Go!

　　Touch your nose, then snap your fingers, then tickle your arm, then touch the floor. Go!

5　Eat soup, then kiss your hand, then pull your ear, then touch your knee, then puff out your cheeks. Go!

　　Hit your knee, then stamp your foot, then touch your nose, then stick out your tongue, then snap your fingers. Go!

　　Tickle your arm, then touch the floor, then touch the floor, then tap your head, then bend your elbow, then rub your eye. Go!

6　Touch your eyebrow, then rub your nose, then stick out your tongue, then rub your eye, then hammer a nail, then clap your hands. Go!

　　Bend your elbow, then throw a ball, then eat soup, then rub your eye, then hit your knee, then kick a ball. Go!

　　Scratch your head, then rub your nose, then touch your knee, then pull your ear, then hammer a nail, then throw a ball. Go!

content. They differ only in the sequence of presentation of the commands. The test begins with the presentation of the first 1-credit instruction. If the child successfully completes this task, 1 point credit is reported on the score sheet (Table 3-4), and the second and third 1-point instructions are presented. The examiner then proceeds to the 3 2-point instructions, the 3-point instructions, etc. In order for credit to be given, the *total* instruction must be carried out in the *exact same sequence* as presented. No partial credit is given. The exami-

Table 3-4   Compliance with Serial Verbal
Instructions — Score Sheet

2. Compliance with Serial Verbal Instructions					
Discontinue after failure of all 3 sequences at the same level.					
Level	Points			Subtotal	
1	1	1	1	3	
					3
2	2	2	2	6	Form A B C
					9
3	3	3	3	9	
					18
4	4	4	4	12	
					30
5	5	5	5	15	
					45
6	6	6	6	18	
					63
					Total Score

nation is discontinued when the child fails all 3 items at the same level. The total score is then calculated on the score sheet (Table 3-4). The normative data (Table 3-5) are used only to ascertain whether or not a child's initial scores are in the normal range. For simplicity, the raw scores only are used for assessing the effects of psychostimulant medication.

When presenting the longer sequences (especially at the 5- and 6-item levels), the examiner may have some difficulty ascertaining whether the child is executing successfully the

Table 3-5   Compliance with Serial Verbal Instructions (Gardner)

	Normative Data — Mean and Standard Deviations					
	Boys			Girls		
Age	*N*	*Mean*	*SD*	*N*	*Mean*	*SD*
5-5½	9	10.33	3.20	6	10.50	3.10
5½-6	13	12.69	4.18	10	10.10	2.43
6-6½	18	13.22	4.25	13	11.85	2.68
6½-7	27	13.37	4.24	17	13.06	2.90
7-7½	23	14.35	4.31	17	14.24	4.94
7½-8	25	16.32	4.33	25	16.76	5.91
8-8½	31	17.00	5.15	25	15.64	4.72
8½-9	25	15.92	5.85	23	15.70	4.31
9-9½	24	16.46	4.68	20	16.25	4.28
9½-10	25	17.32	4.25	14	14.07	3.15
10-10½	17	20.00	5.36	21	18.24	5.15
10½-11	23	19.30	4.43	16	18.50	3.32
11-11½	14	20.86	8.26	16	20.31	6.38
11½-12	17	18.94	5.98	8	21.00	5.36
12-12½	9	25.56	6.50	11	21.91	5.71
12½-13	8	18.75	7.14	9	22.11	8.45
13-13½	14	21.07	4.37	6	25.17	10.78
13½-14	5	21.80	6.40	7	25.57	4.14
14-14½	4	21.75	5.89	5	24.80	3.92
14½-15	2	22.00	4.00	3	20.00	5.89
15-15½	5	26.20	4.75	4	31.75	13.01
15½-16	5	25.20	2.99	4	21.25	3.11

task. The reason for this is that the examiner is required to observe both the child and the instruction sheet at the same time, or to quickly look back and forth between the child and the instruction sheet. If, in the course of such assessment, the examiner is not certain whether or not the child did indeed successfully execute the task, a new task of the same length should be presented by random selection of items from the various levels.

3. WISC-R: Digit Span, Digits Forward (Wechsler, Gardner)   When administering the Digits Forward section of the Digit Span subtest of the *Wechsler Intelligence Scale for Children Revised* (WISC-R) (D. Wechsler, 1974), the child is presented with progressively longer numerical sequences and is asked to repeat them immediately after presentation. The instrument assesses auditory concentration and short-term auditory sequential memory. Wechsler's criteria for obtaining the raw score are utilized. However, the Wechsler scoring system does not permit the examiner to obtain separate scaled scores for the Digits Forward and Digits Backward sections. There are drawbacks to the failure to make this differentiation in that most children do not form an internalized mental image of the numbers when performing the Digits Forward task but do so with the Digits Backward task. When performing the latter they usually scan the mentally visualized sequences and verbalize the numbers while doing so. Accordingly, children with visual processing impairments may do poorly on the Digits Backward section of the test. However, their high score on the Digits Forward section may so counterbalance the low score on the Digits Backward that they may appear to perform normally. The Digits Backward impairment thereby gets "buried" and undetected. In order to correct this defect of the Digit Span test, my assistants and I have administered the subtest to normal children, boys and girls ages 5 - 16, and have presented these findings as 2 separate subtests. Means, standard deviations, and percentile ranks are presented that enable the examiner to ascertain exactly the degree of abnormality in each of the 2 categories. The normative Digits Forward data are presented in Table 3-6 (R.A. Gardner, 1979 and 1981).

For the purposes of the PMAB, only the raw scores are utilized. Also, for the purposes of the PMAB 2 alternative forms of the Digits Forward sequences have been prepared. At each level the same numbers utilized in the Wechsler scale are used. However, they have been randomized to provide alternative sequences. Wechsler's original numerical sequences have been designated Form 3A. The alternative forms have been designated Forms 3B and 3C.

4. WISC-R: Digit Span, Digits Backward (Wechsler, Gardner)   When administering the Digits Backward section of the Digit Span subtest of the WISC-R, the child is asked to repeat the presented sequences in reverse order. The instrument assesses the same functions as the Digits Forward section, namely, auditory attention and short-term auditory sequential memory. However, it also assesses a type of short-term visual sequential memory because most (but not all) patients form an internal image of the numerical sequence, and then scan it both forward and backward, before verbalizing the sequence in reverse. Accordingly, it can be considered to assess a type of short-term visual sequential memory, visual concentration, and visual scanning. It is because of this extra function that this examiner separated the Digits Forward and Digits Backward sections into two separate tests.

The original Wechsler numerical sequences are designated Form 4A and are administered in accordance with the Wechsler criteria for obtaining the raw score. This examiner's standardized data is utilized for obtaining the child's score on this instrument. Again, 2 alternative forms of the same numerical sequences have been prepared. At each level the same

Table 3-6   The Digits Forward Section of the WISC-R
Normative Data — Means and Standard Deviations

Digit Span — Digits Forward for Boys

Age	N	Mean	S.D.
5-0 to 5-5	26	3.27	1.31
5-6 to 5-11	29	4.03	1.70
6-0 to 6-5	33	4.67	1.93
6-6 to 6-11	43	4.88	1.73
7-0 to 7-5	45	5.18	1.86
7-6 to 7-11	53	5.47	1.99
8-0 to 8-5	36	5.81	2.05
8-6 to 8-11	47	6.17	2.32
9-0 to 9-5	38	6.21	1.77
9-6 to 9-11	34	6.85	2.22
10-0 to 10-5	29	5.97	1.78
10-6 to 10-11	22	7.18	2.02
11-0 to 11-5	34	7.00	2.10
11-6 to 11-11	35	7.06	1.91
12-0 to 12-5	35	7.80	1.94
12-6 to 12-11	40	7.88	2.04
13-0 to 13-5	51	7.71	2.12
13-6 to 13-11	38	8.29	2.00
14-0 to 14-5	35	7.89	2.04
14-6 to 14-11	36	7.56	1.98
15-0 to 15-5	27	7.26	2.49
15-6 to 15-11	16	7.06	2.02
	782		

Digit Span — Digits Forward for Girls

Age	N	Mean	S.D.
5-0 to 5-5	27	3.48	1.19
5-6 to 5-11	22	4.86	1.70
6-0 to 6-5	30	4.60	1.43
6-6 to 6-11	36	4.97	1.84
7-0 to 7-5	43	5.26	1.65
7-6 to 7-11	42	5.86	1.76
8-0 to 8-5	37	6.19	1.93
8-6 to 8-11	51	6.61	1.80
9-0 to 9-5	38	6.42	2.09
9-6 to 9-11	28	7.54	2.96
10-0 to 10-5	30	7.10	1.60
10-6 to 10-11	29	7.00	1.85
11-0 to 11-5	52	6.77	1.95
11-6 to 11-11	36	7.17	1.93
12-0 to 12-5	37	7.43	1.88
12-6 to 12-11	47	7.85	1.90
13-0 to 13-5	42	8.12	2.27
13-6 to 13-11	36	8.61	2.18
14-0 to 14-5	36	7.25	1.93
14-6 to 14-11	34	7.88	1.53
15-0 to 15-5	25	8.08	2.27
15-6 to 15-11	27	7.56	1.99
	785		

Reprinted from Gardner, R.A. (1979), *The Objective Diagnosis of Minimal Brain Dysfunction*. Cresskill, New Jersey: Creative Therapeutics.

WISC-R
Digit Span, Digits Forward

<u>Form 3A</u>

Item	Trial 1	Trial 2
1.	3-8-6	6-1-2
2.	3-4-1-7	6-1-5-8
3.	8-4-2-3-9	5-2-1-8-6
4.	3-8-9-1-7-4	7-9-6-4-8-3
5.	5-1-7-4-2-3-8	9-8-5-2-1-6-3
6.	1-6-4-5-9-7-6-3	2-9-7-6-3-1-5-4
7.	5-3-8-7-1-2-4-6-9	4-2-6-9-1-7-8-3-5

<u>Form 3B</u>

Item	Trial 1	Trial 2
1.	6-8-3	1-6-2
2.	7-3-4-1	5-1-8-6
3.	2-9-3-4-8	1-6-8-2-5
4.	7-3-9-8-4-1	4-6-8-9-3-7
5.	8-3-4-2-1-5-7	5-3-6-2-8-1-9
6.	6-4-5-7-6-1-3-9	2-3-5-1-4-9-7-6
7.	3-7-9-8-4-1-5-2-6	6-8-3-2-5-9-4-1-7

<u>Form 3C</u>

Item	Trial 1	Trial 2
1.	8-3-6	2-6-1
2.	1-7-4-3	8-6-1-5
3.	4-9-8-3-2	2-6-5-8-1
4.	7-4-1-9-8-3	4-9-6-7-3-8
5.	8-1-7-2-5-3-4	1-6-5-8-2-3-9
6.	4-6-1-7-3-6-9-5	6-4-9-1-3-2-7-5
7.	2-7-5-3-8-6-4-9-1	7-3-4-9-6-1-2-5-8

WISC-R
Digit Span, Digits Backward

Form 4A

Item	Trial 1	Trial 2
1.	2-5	6-3
2.	5-7-4	2-5-9
3.	7-2-9-6	8-4-9-3
4.	4-1-3-5-7	9-7-8-5-2
5.	1-6-5-2-9-8	3-6-7-1-9-4
6.	8-5-9-2-3-4-2	4-5-7-9-2-8-1
7.	6-9-1-6-3-2-5-8	3-1-7-9-5-4-8-2

Form 4B

Item	Trial 1	Trial 2
1.	5-2	3-6
2.	5-4-7	9-2-5
3.	6-2-7-9	4-3-9-8
4.	3-5-4-7-1	7-5-2-8-9
5.	9-1-5-2-8-6	4-9-3-7-1-6
6.	2-9-5-3-8-2-4	5-9-2-8-7-4-1
7.	6-2-1-5-3-8-9-6	8-2-7-9-1-5-3-9

Form 4C

Item	Trial 1	Trial 2
1.	2-5	6-3
2.	7-4-5	5-9-2
3.	2-9-7-6	4-9-8-3
4.	7-3-5-1-4	2-8-5-7-9
5.	5-9-8-2-6-1	7-3-6-4-8-1
6.	4-8-2-9-3-5-2	8-5-2-7-1-9-4
7.	1-8-2-6-9-5-6-3	4-9-1-3-8-7-2-5

numbers are used as when the Wechsler scale is utilized; however, they are presented in alternative, randomized sequences. These alternative forms have been designated Forms 4B and 4C. Normative data for Digits Backward are presented in Table 3-7.

5. The Steadiness Tester (Gardner et al.) When utilizing this instrument the child is asked to hold a stylus in a hole as steadily as possible. Each time the stylus touches the hole's perimeter, a buzzer sounds and a timer records the total duration of contact time (Figure 3-2). Three 60-second trials are administered. The instrument assesses hyperactivity and visual attention-sustaining capacity. Normative data (Table 3-8) obtained by this examiner are utilized in ascertaining the child's score. The instrument does not lend itself to the presentation of alternative forms of administration. Accordingly, the same mode of presentation is utilized during the 3 practice trials as well as the 6 trials used in the period of drug assessment.

6. Cancellation of Rapidly Recurring Target Figures (Rudel et al.) When administering this instrument, the child is presented with a sheet of paper (Form 6A) on the top of which is the model numerical sequence 592. Below is an array of 140 3-digit numbers, all of which begin with the number 5. Fourteen of the 3-digit numbers are 592s and the other 136 are not. The child is asked to place a cross over all numerical sequences that are identical to the model and leave alone all those that are not. The child is scored both with regard to the number of errors made (both omission and comission) as well as the time taken to complete the task. Erasing is permitted. The instrument assesses visual attention, short-term visual memory, and visual discrimination. The original Rudel et al. (1978) format is designated Form 6A. Two other renditions have been prepared. These include the exact same numerical

Table 3-7 The Digits Backward Section of the WISC-R
Normative Data—Means and Standard Deviations

Digit Span—Digits Backward for Boys				Digit Span—Digits Backward for Girls			
Age	N	Mean	S.D.	Age	N	Mean	S.D.
5-0 to 5-5	26	1.69	1.12	5-0 to 5-5	27	1.22	1.36
5-6 to 5-11	29	1.66	1.47	5-6 to 5-11	22	1.36	1.09
6-0 to 6-5	33	2.48	1.44	6-0 to 6-5	30	2.67	1.42
6-6 to 6-11	43	3.23	1.17	6-6 to 6-11	36	3.47	1.13
7-0 to 7-5	45	3.62	1.39	7-0 to 7-5	43	3.72	1.47
7-6 to 7-11	53	3.87	1.00	7-6 to 7-11	42	3.76	1.25
8-0 to 8-5	36	3.69	1.43	8-0 to 8-5	37	3.97	1.17
8-6 to 8-11	47	3.85	1.22	8-6 to 8-11	51	4.02	1.39
9-0 to 9-5	38	4.26	1.27	9-0 to 9-5	38	4.05	1.63
9-6 to 9-11	34	4.82	2.05	9-6 to 9-11	28	4.79	1.50
10-0 to 10-5	29	4.31	1.37	10-0 to 10-5	30	4.53	1.50
10-6 to 10-11	22	6.09	2.07	10-6 to 10-11	29	5.00	1.67
11-0 to 11-5	34	5.09	1.75	11-0 to 11-5	52	5.35	1.82
11-6 to 11-11	35	4.89	1.37	11-6 to 11-11	36	5.72	2.16
12-0 to 12-5	35	5.14	1.88	12-0 to 12-5	37	5.30	1.68
12-6 to 12-11	40	5.43	1.75	12-6 to 12-11	47	5.68	1.75
13-0 to 13-5	51	5.22	1.85	13-0 to 13-5	42	5.74	1.68
13-6 to 13-11	38	5.82	2.14	13-6 to 13-11	36	5.31	1.85
14-0 to 14-5	35	4.68	1.54	14-0 to 14-5	36	5.08	1.90
14-6 to 14-11	36	5.17	1.59	14-6 to 14-11	34	6.12	2.52
15-0 to 15-5	27	4.52	1.58	15-0 to 15-5	25	5.72	1.37
15-6 to 15-11	16	5.13	1.36	15-6 to 15-11	27	6.26	2.16
	782				785		

Reprinted from Gardner, R.A. (1979), *The Objective Diagnosis of Minimal Brain Dysfunction.* Cresskill, New Jersey: Creative Therapeutics.

Figure 3-2 Steadiness Tester: Child and Examiner Correctly Positioned for Testing

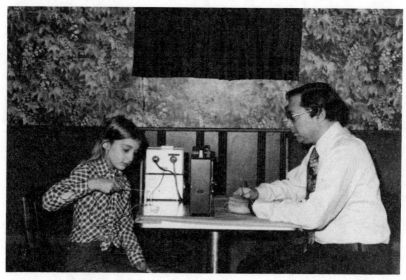

sequences presented in another randomization. These have been designated Forms 6B and 6C. Normative data are to be found in Table 3-9.

7. The Recognition Subtest of The Reversals Frequency Test (Gardner)   When utilizing this instrument, the child is presented with a sheet of paper on which are an array of numbers and letters, some of which are correctly oriented and others are printed in mirror image orientation (Form 7). The child is asked to place a cross over all incorrectly oriented numbers and letters. There is no time limit and erasing *is* permitted. The examiner records on the test sheet the total number of errors, both omission and commission. The instrument assesses long-term visual memory for letter and number orientation. This examiner's normative data (Table 3-10) are used for scoring. This is another test that does not lend itself well to the preparation of 3 different forms. Accordingly, the same instrument is presented during the practice phase as well as the drug-assessment phase of the study.

Table 3-8   Steadiness Tester — Total Touch Time
Normative Data — Means and Standard Deviations

Age	N	Mean	S.D.	Age	N	Mean	S.D.
Normal Boys				Normal Girls			
5-0 to 5-11	26	39.03	20.95	5-0 to 5-11	27	30.37	22.63
6-0 to 6-11	30	25.45	16.59	6-0 to 6-11	29	22.05	14.40
7-0 to 7-11	27	13.93	9.53	7-0 to 7-11	25	13.77	9.74
8-0 to 8-11	28	8.23	6.06	8-0 to 8-11	27	5.77	5.77
9-0 to 9-11	27	10.43	7.18	9-0 to 9-11	25	5.75	5.54
10-0 to 10-11	28	8.80	7.33	10-0 to 10-11	25	5.01	3.72
11-0 to 11-11	25	3.97	3.78	11-0 to 11-11	25	2.10	1.88
12-0 to 12-11	26	5.40	5.79	12-0 to 12-11	25	1.87	1.47
13-0 to 13-11	27	3.77	3.25	13-0 to 13-11	25	1.17	1.05
14-0 to 14-11	12	4.99	5.83	14-0 to 14-11	11	3.25	2.86
	256				244		

Reprinted from Gardner, R.A. (1979), *The Objective Diagnosis of Minimal Brain Dysfunction.*
Cresskill, New Jersey: Creative Therapeutics.

Form 6A

592

569	562	598	561	591	564	563	591	569	561
564	561	592	599	562	594	591	562	598	592
599	593	563	564	591	598	562	564	569	599
563	599	594	569	561	591	592	599	592	564
561	564	591	562	599	599	561	569	598	594
594	592	563	569	594	564	594	599	561	563
569	562	569	599	598	563	591	564	599	592
563	592	561	563	591	561	569	598	562	569
562	591	594	564	592	563	599	592	599	591
598	561	592	599	562	594	564	562	563	598
564	563	599	598	594	569	592	561	599	562
598	592	569	591	564	562	594	598	594	591
561	563	564	562	592	598	563	562	592	564
569	591	598	594	561	569	591	594	561	563

Form 6B

592

562	591	592	564	593	599	593	563	564	591
598	562	564	569	599	564	563	592	598	594
563	599	592	599	591	562	594	598	594	591
564	563	591	569	561	564	561	592	599	562
569	591	594	561	563	594	591	562	598	592
598	592	569	591	564	563	599	594	569	561
594	592	563	569	594	564	594	599	561	563
569	562	569	593	598	561	564	591	562	599
563	594	564	599	592	598	563	562	592	564
591	564	599	592	564	593	561	569	598	594
598	561	592	599	562	594	564	562	563	598
569	591	598	594	561	563	592	561	563	591
569	592	561	599	562	561	562	598	562	569
561	563	564	562	592	569	562	598	561	591

Form 6C

592

598	562	564	569	599	564	563	591	569	561
564	594	599	561	563	569	592	561	599	562
564	563	592	598	594	569	591	598	594	561
562	591	592	564	592	562	594	598	594	591
599	593	563	564	591	598	563	562	592	564
561	564	591	562	599	569	562	598	561	591
563	592	564	599	562	561	593	598	562	569
563	598	561	563	591	569	562	569	592	598
561	563	564	562	592	563	599	594	569	561
594	564	562	563	598	593	561	569	598	594
598	561	592	599	562	594	562	563	569	594
569	591	594	561	563	591	598	599	592	564
564	561	592	599	562	594	591	562	598	592
598	592	569	591	564	563	599	592	599	591

Table 3-9   Cancellation of Rapidly Recurring Target Figures (Rudel et al.)

			Time	
		592		
Age	Mean	S.D. (rounded off)	Mean	S.D.
4-5	13	(4)	—	—
6-7	6	(3)	200.76	(81.51)
8-9	2	(2)	116.00	(33.71)
10-11	2	(2)	90.70	(24.66)
12-13	2	(2)	67.13	(15.76)

Reprinted with permission of Rita Rudel, Ph.D., Martha Denckla, M.D., and Melinda Broman, Ph.D.

Form 7

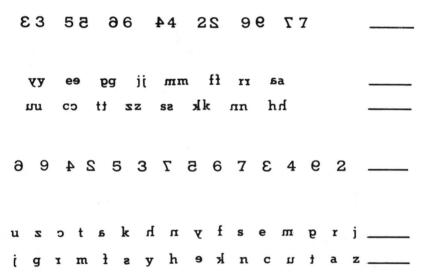

Table 3-10 The Recognition Subtest of
The Reversals Frequency Test (Gardner)
Normative Data — Means and Standard Deviations

Age	Boys			Girls		
	N	Mean	S.D.	N	Mean	S.D.
5-0 to 5-11	25	23.76	11.11	28	21.20	10.25
6-0 to 6-11	28	18.54	11.52	31	13.00	9.49
7-0 to 7-11	25	8.16	5.31	25	5.64	6.48
8-0 to 8-11	26	3.73	4.07	27	2.63	2.80
9-0 to 9-11	27	3.15	3.03	25	2.24	2.22
10-0 to 10-11	30	2.07	2.73	27	1.74	1.68
11-0 to 11-11	26	2.81	3.12	25	2.36	2.78
12-0 to 12-11	25	1.56	1.66	25	1.36	1.68
13-0 to 13-11	27	1.96	2.24	25	1.08	1.35
14-0 to 14-11	12	2.42	2.06	11	1.20	1.60
	251			249		

Reprinted from Gardner, R.A. (1978), *The Reversals Frequency Test.* Cresskill, New Jersey: Creative Therapeutics.

Gardner, R.A. (1979), *The Objective Diagnosis of Minimal Brain Dysfunction.* Cresskill, New Jersey: Creative Therapeutics.

8. WISC-R: Block Design (Wechsler) When utilizing the Block Design subtest of the WISC-R (D. Wechsler, 1974), the child is presented with a collection blocks on each facet of which are varying red and white designs. The child is asked to reproduce with the blocks designs presented on a series of picture cards. The instrument assesses visual-motor organization, visual analysis, visual-motor synthesis, and visual-motor Gestalt. The original Wechsler presentation has been designated Form 8A. When administering Form 8A, the examiner should hold the booklet of printed designs in such a way that the spiral top is under his or her thumb. This is designated the *north* orientation. Three other modes of presentation of the design booklet are possible, namely, east, south, and west. The east presentation is accomplished by the examiner's holding the design booklet with his or her thumb at the east position on the page. Similarly, the south and west positions provide the opportunity for additional modes of presentation. For the purposes of the PMAB the east mode of presentation is designated Form 8B and the south mode of presentation Form 8C. In this way an attempt is made to obviate the practice effect. The same scoring criteria are utilized for all 3 modes of presentation. For the purposes of the PMAB the *raw scores* rather than the scaled scores are used.

9. The Assembly Section of the Purdue Pegboard (Lafayette Instrument Co., Gardner) The Purdue Pegboard consists of 2 parallel rows of 25 holes in each row. Pegs, collars, and washers are located in 4 cups at the top of the board. In the assembly section (Figure 3-3) the child is asked to form

Figure 3-3 The Assembly Section of the Purdue Pegboard

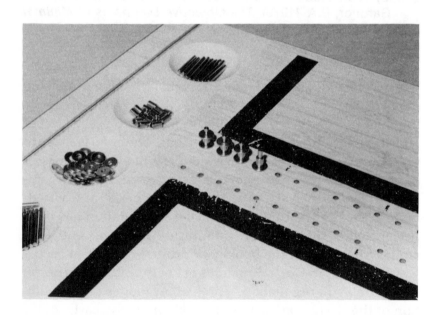

"assemblies" consisting of a peg, a washer, a collar, and another washer as rapidly as possible. The instrument assesses fine motor coordination and visual-motor coordination. The instrument has been standardized for children by this examiner, whose normative data is utilized for scoring. Four points credits is given for each assembly completed in the 60-seconds alloted for the test. Partial credit (1, 2, or 3 points) is awarded for uncompleted assemblies. This is another one of the PMAB tests that does not lend itself well to the preparation of alternative equivalent forms. Accordingly, the same administration technique is utilized during the 3 practice trials as well as the 6-trial drug study. Normative data (R.A. Gardner, 1979) are presented in Table 3-11.

10. Developmental Test of Visual-Motor Integration (Beery and Buktenica)   When administering this instrument, the child is asked to copy as accurately as possible a series of model geometric patterns. The instrument assesses visual-motor coordination, visual discrimination, and visual Gestalt. Children with constructional dyspraxia are likely to perform poorly. Strict scoring criteria are utilized with 1 point credit being given if the copy is correct in accordance with specific scoring criteria for that particular pattern. No credit is given if the copy does not satisfy the scoring criteria. Erasing is *not* permitted. This is another one of the PMAB tests that does not lend itself to the preparation of alternative forms. Accordingly, the same method of presentation is utilized throughout the 3 practice testing periods as well as the 6 drug-assessment presentations.

CONCLUDING COMMENTS

I have presented here in detail *The Psychostimulant Medication Assessment Battery*. First, certain GMBDS deficits that were reported in the literature to be improved by psychostimulant

Table 3-11   The Assembly Section of The Purdue Pegboard
(Lafayette Instrument Co., Gardner)
Normative Data — Means and Standard Deviations

Age	Boys			Girls		
	N	Mean	S.D.	N	Mean	S.D.
5-0 to 5-5	30	14.10	3.29	30	14.70	2.55
5-6 to 5-11	30	15.57	3.56	30	14.37	4.02
6-0 to 6-5	30	15.93	2.94	30	18.03	3.54
6-6 to 6-11	30	19.20	3.84	30	20.63	4.27
7-0 to 7-5	30	19.23	4.95	30	19.77	4.49
7-6 to 7-11	30	20.40	4.10	30	20.20	4.61
8-0 to 8-5	30	23.20	3.80	30	21.93	4.31
8-6 to 8-11	30	24.47	5.35	30	24.50	5.83
9-0 to 9-5	30	24.57	3.75	30	24.97	6.81
9-6 to 9-11	30	27.37	4.55	30	29.07	6.01
10-0 to 10-5	30	26.37	6.15	30	27.90	5.10
10-6 to 10-11	30	28.17	5.38	30	31.70	6.02
11-0 to 11-5	30	29.53	6.19	30	32.77	5.50
11-6 to 11-11	30	31.33	5.19	30	33.47	7.24
12-0 to 12-5	30	31.13	5.78	30	34.57	5.20
12-6 to 12-11	30	30.13	6.08	30	34.70	7.52
13-0 to 13-5	40	33.73	5.00	40	34.85	5.57
13-6 to 13-11	30	34.57	5.88	32	37.40	5.34
14-0 to 14-5	30	33.97	6.58	30	36.43	6.76
14-6 to 14-11	30	31.37	7.24	30	34.17	6.62
15-0 to 15-5	30	32.20	6.21	28	36.89	7.75
15-6 to 15-11	23	33.04	6.24	31	37.35	8.24
	663			671		

Reprinted from Gardner, R.A. (1979), *The Objective Diagnosis of Minimal Brain Dysfunction.* Cresskill, New Jersey: Creative Therapeutics.

medication were selected: Specifically, the following deficits were selected; attention-sustaining impairment (ADD), hyperactivity, visual-perceptual impairment, and fine motor coordination deficit. Then, tests were selected that specifically assess for the presence of the aforementioned deficits. Next, an attempt was made to ascertain whether psychostimulant medication would indeed improve a child's performance on these tests when a deficit was present. If it was found that one or more of the tests were indeed sensitive to psychostimulant medication, then an attempt would be made to determine whether the instrument could be used for monitoring drug medication. In this chapter the basic battery has been described. In the next chapter I will discuss the scores obtained from a series of children and the implications of my findings, not only for the specific purposes of the study but for my theory on the causes of GMBDS.

FOUR

Results of the Study and Implications for the Theory

INTRODUCTORY COMMENTS

Here I present the findings of the first 9 patients who were administered the PMAB. All of them were children who manifested one or more signs and/or symptoms of GMBDS on a clinical basis. In addition, 7 of the 9 (with the exception of patients #7 and #9) manifested abnormal scores on the Steadiness Tester (using the criteria described in Chapter Three), suggesting strongly they were hyperactive. And 7 of them (again with the exception of patients #7 and #9) exhibited deficiencies in 1 or more of the other tests of the PMAB.

All of the patients were boys. This is no surprise in that about 90+% of all the GMBDS patients referred to me are males. I believe the traditional ratio of 3–4 boys to every girl is low. I believe that the reason for the preponderance of boys over girls relates to a number of factors. First, males are indeed the weaker sex. The best estimates are that there are about 200 male embryos to every 100 female embryos. The intrauterine death rate of males is far greater than that of females, so much so that at the time of birth the ratio of males to females is approximately 106 to 100. And the post-natal death rate of males is also greater than that of females. In fact, the death rate for most diseases (with the exception of diseases of the breasts and female genitalia) is higher in males than females. The result is that females in just about every country live longer than males—in many countries as much as 8 to 9 years longer. The result is that the populations of old-age homes are predominantly female.

There is another factor that contributes to the predominance of males over females in the GMBDS population referred for treatment. This relates to the hyperactivity symptom. As mentioned, boys represent the survivors of the warriors, hunters, and food gatherers; in contrast, females, over the span of evolution, were traditionally the child rearers. The more active and assertive men were likely to be more successful as warriors and hunters. In fact, considering the predatory nature of the world and the murderous competition that was ubiquitous throughout mankind's history it is reasonable to assume that the passive, meek, and less assertive were more likely to be killed and their genes were less likely to have been transmitted to their descendents. Speak to nurses and attendants in a nursery for newborn infants. They will tell you that the boys are typically more active and demanding, whereas the girls are usually more passive and compliant. Speak to grade-school teachers. They too will tell you that the boys are much more active than the girls, much more self-assertive, and in general "tougher customers."

Some believe that these differences are environmentally induced. I do not deny that there may be some environmental factors that contribute to this difference. However, to deny the genetic programming is to deny the realities of history and evolution. When we take these hunters and warriors and place them in a school—where they are asked to sit still 5 to 6 hours a day—we are asking for trouble. Some societies (such as in Japan and Germany) are more successful in repressing their youngsters. In the United States we are generally quite liberal regarding child rearing and active behavior is less suppressed. I am not precluding the genetic factors, only pointing out that environmental influences can certainly suppress hyperactive behavior to some degree.

One other factor that may be contributing to the predominance of males in my practice may relate to the fact that as a male I am more likely to get male patients, with parents preferring to send their female children and adolescents to female therapists. In some cases this may be unfortunate because a male therapist would be preferable, e.g., situations in which the youngster's father is no longer in the home, has been cruel and rejecting, or otherwise has served as a poor role model.

Of the 9 children studied 7 were on Ritalin and 2 (patients #6 and #8) were on Dexedrine. My experience has been that there is very little difference in the effectiveness of these 2 medications. I generally start on Ritalin (methylphenidate) and, if not significantly successful, I will then switch to Dexedrine (dextroamphatamine sulfate). I rarely use Cylert (pemoline). My reason for this is that it generally takes 7 to 10 days before one can see results. With Ritalin and Dexedrine results can generally be observed in 30-60 minutes. The time lag with Cylert not only results in time lost regarding getting the child to optimum levels, but makes it practically impossible to monitor the drug with instruments such as the Steadiness Tester and other potential assessment instruments utilized in this study. The 2 patients who were on Dexedrine were those who originally showed little if any response to Ritalin. My main reason for choosing Ritalin first is that in recent years there appears to be less concern on the part of pharmacists and drug control agencies regarding prescribing

Ritalin. Because Dexedrine ("speed") is much more likely to find its way into the illicit drug market, prescribing it may involve more forms to be filled out, red tape, delay, and questioning.

DISCUSSION OF RESULTS

Steven B. (Patient #1)

Steven B. was 12 years old and in the 7th grade when he was referred by his school because of agitation and disruptive behavior in the classroom. He was defiant of his teachers and would often direct profanities against them. On other occasions he was passive-aggressive and obstructionistic in the classroom. His academic curiosity and motivation were seriously impaired, so that he was getting very low grades even though considered to be of above average intelligence. There were significant marital problems in the home and the parents were continually fighting. However, the question of divorce never entered either of their minds; so enmeshed were they in their sadomasochistic relationship.

Ritalin was found to be effective in improving Steven's behavior in the classroom in that he became more cooperative and less hyperactive. Clinically, a dose of 10 mg. in the morning and at noon was found to be optimum. As can be seen from Table 4-1 the average Steadiness Tester score for boys his age is 5.4 seconds. Steven's first score was 50 seconds and his scores on 2 further practice trials were 84.0 and 100.8 seconds. The figures in the drug-free/post-drug assessment trials strongly suggest that the Steadiness Tester is a sensitive indicator of Ritalin efficacy. This was confirmed by statistical analysis of the data obtained in the 6 drug trials ($p < .001$). It is possible that Steven's poor performance on the Steadiness Tester was related to a visual concentration deficit in that the child must attend visually to the task to insure that the stylus

Table 4-1 Psychostimulant Medication Assessment Battery Tabulation of Data

Assessment Instrument	Norm.	Score	Defic.	Practice Trials	Drug Assessment Trials 1 Drug free	2 Post drug	3 Drug free	4 Post drug	5 Drug free	6 Post drug	p
1. Word Span	31.8	A 19	Yes	A 20	A 19	C 28	B 19	A 37	C 33	B 32	NS
2. Compliance with Serial Verbal Instructions	25.5	A 22	No	A 20	A 12	C 22	B 18	A 26	C 26	B 18	NS
3. Digit Span Digits Forward (WISC-R)	7.8	A 9	No	A 6	A 5	C 8	B 2	A 8	C 5	B 6	<.10 NS
4. Digit Span Digits Backward (WISC-R)	5.1	A 4	No	A 4	A 6	C 7	B 4	A 8	C 6	B 9	<.01
5. Steadiness Tester	5.4"	A 50"	Yes	A 84.0" 100.8"	A 128.8"	A 4.1'"	A 165.5"	A 13"	A 120.1"	A 5.2"	<.001
6. Cancellation of Rapidly Recurring Target Figures	2±2E 67±15"	A 5E 230"	Yes / Yes	A 6E 142" 7E 148"	A 9E 123"	A HE 115"	B 6E 82"	A 0E 32"	C 12E 79"	B 1E 33"	NS <.10 NS
7. Reversals Frequency Test, Recognition	1.56	A 12	Yes	A 5	A 8	A 1	A 7	A 0	A 0	A 1	NS
8. Block Design (WISC-R)	SS10 RS32%	A SS9 RS28	No	A SS9 RS26 SS7 RS21	A SS10 RS44 SS9 RS44	C SS10 RS44	B SS14 RS50	SS15 RS52	C SS17 RS52	B SS16 RS56	NS
9. Purdue Pegboard	50% 29	A <10% 17	Yes	A <10% 7 <20% 8	A <10% 16	A <10% 12	A <10% 9	A <10% 16	A <10% 16	B <10% 20	NS
10. Development Test of Visual-Motor Integration	50% 19.5"	A 32% 18	No	A 19% 12 5% 12	A 63% 5	A 42% 16	A 21% 15	A 32% 18	A 16% 14	A 55% 20	NS

Name **Steven B (#1)** Age **12** years **5** months Sex **M** Drug **RITALIN** Dose **10 Mg** does not touch the perimeter of the hole. Steven also did poorly on both sections (number of errors and time to perform the task) of the Cancellation of Rapidly Recurring Target Figures test and his poor performance persisted throughout the practice trials. However, analysis of the data obtained from the 6 drug-free/post-drug trials does not reveal strong evidence that Ritalin had produced improvement in Steven's performance on this instrument ($p < .10$). The findings here suggest that Ritalin's effect in improving Steven's performance on the Steadiness Tester was less likely related to a visual concentration improvement than to its effect on his hyperactivity.

The first 4 tests of the PMAB assess primarily auditory attention (as opposed to visual attention). Of these tests only The Word Span Test was in the abnormal range at the outset. However, an attempt was made to ascertain whether all 4 of these instruments would be Ritalin sensitive. The data indicates that Ritalin did not improve Steven's score on The Word Span Test, the one that showed a deficient score. Nor did it affect his score on the Compliance with Serial Verbal Instructions test. Improvement on Digits Forward was found to be present at the $p < .10$ level, which was not considered to be significant. On Digits Backward, however, there was improvement at the $p < .01$ level. This improvement, however, was of a score that was already within the normal range.

On the Recognition section of the Reversals Frequency Test a deficiency was found, but Steven's improvement was not found to be related to Ritalin. I suspect that the improvement was related to the practice effect. Steven's scaled score on the Block Design subtest of the WISC-R was 9, i.e. the lower end of the normal range. Although his score was normal, attempts were made to determine whether this instrument was Ritalin sensitive. Using *raw scores* for statistical analysis there were no significant differences between Steven's drug-free and post-drug scores. There was, however, a general trend toward improved Block Design performance over the course of the study, suggesting that presenting the sample cards in different orientations did not serve well to obviate the practice effect.

Steven exhibited a deficiency on the Purdue Pegboard—suggesting a fine motor coordination problem. Analysis of his data did not indicate Ritalin sensitivity. Furthermore, examination of the data reveals that there was no improvement over the course of the study—suggesting that the practice effect was not a contaminant to this conclusion.

On the Developmental Test of Visual-Motor Integration Steven's initial score was 18 points (32nd percentile). A score of 19.5 is at the 50th percentile level. Accordingly, no impairment was considered to be present. However, during the 2 practice trials he scored at the 1 and 5 percentile levels. These lowered levels of performance reflected the clinically observed lack of commitment and cooperation and cannot be considered to negate the original normal score. Accordingly, no deficiency was considered to be present. An attempt was still made to ascertain whether his performance on this test was Ritalin sensitive. The analysis of the data revealed no significant differences between post-drug and drug-free trials.

My final conclusion with regard to Steven is that Steadiness Tester scores proved Ritalin sensitive at the $p < .001$ level and the Digits Backward test proved sensitive at the $p < .01$ level. None of the other 8 instruments of the PMAB proved Ritalin sensitive.

Brian W. (Patient #2)

This 13-year-old boy was referred because of school difficulties, especially in the learning area. He was distractable in the classroom and was considered to have an attention-deficit disorder. He was also hyperactive and auditory perceptual problems were described. When frustrated, he would have violent temper outbursts, during which times he would kick walls and furniture. On both a clinical basis and via the utilization of the Steadiness Tester it was found that his optimum Ritalin dosage was 25 mg. twice a day. Previous examiners trying 10 and 15 mg. twice a day were not able to say definitely whether or not his behavior was responding to Ritalin. However, when the dose was increased to 25 mg. twice a day there was definite improvement clinically and this was confirmed by both his parents and his teachers.

As can be seen from Table 4-2 Brian did not exhibit any impairments in the first 4 PMAB tests—tests that assess primarily auditory attention. However, even though no deficits were present, drug-free/post-drug assessment trials were administered. There was no evidence that any of these 4 instruments were Ritalin sensitive.

With the Steadiness Tester Brian exhibited definite impairment and this impairment persisted throughout the practice trials. As can be seen from the data obtained during the drug-free/post-drug assessment trials, each of his drug-free scores was higher than each of the post-drug scores. However, statistical analysis of the data did not reveal these improvements to be significant ($p < .10$).

There was no evidence for impairment in the ability to cancel rapidly recurring target figures or in reversals frequency. It was decided not to assess these functions further by utilization of the drug assessment trials.

An impairment was seen on the Block Design subtest of the WISC-R. And this impairment persisted throughout the practice trials. An analysis of the data cofirmed that there was no significant difference between Brian's post-drug and the drug-free scores. Interestingly, whereas Steven B. (Patient #1) exhibited improvement in Block Design over the course of the 6 drug-assessment trials, suggesting practice effect, this was not the case for Brian W. Although there was some variation

Table 4-2 Psychostimulant Medication Assessment Battery Tabulation of Data

Assessment Instrument	Norm.	Score	Defic.	Practice Trials	1 Drug free	2 Post drug	3 Drug free	4 Post drug	5 Drug free	6 Post drug	p
1. Word Span	37.7	A 28	N	A 32 / A 26	A 23	C 37	B 27	A 32	C 42	B 23	NS
2. Compliance with Serial Verbal Instructions	21.8	A 22	N	A	A	A 22	C 22	B 23	A 15	C 18	B 22	NS
3. Digit Span Digits Forward (WISC-R) school 3/83	7.7	A 8	N	A 7	A 12	C 9	B 10	A 12	C 9	B 8	NS
4. Digit Span Digits Backward (WISC-R) school 3/83	5.2	A 6	N	A 7	A 4	C 8	B 6	A 5	C 6	B 7	NS
5. Steadiness Tester	3.7	A 15.8	Y	A 29.3 / A 29.7	A 12.7	A 3.42	A 17.31	A 7.88	A 6.72	A 2.99	<.10 (ns)
6. Cancellation of Rapidly Recurring Target Figures	4 2E / 6'1"/4'28" 60"	A 1 / 60"	N	A	A	C	B	A	C	B	
7. Reversals Frequency Test, Recognition	2.0	A 0	N	A	A	A	A	A	A	A	
8. Block Design (WISC-R) school 3/83	55 / 10 / 15-22	A 55 / 25	Y	A 55 / 23 / 20	A 55 / 45 / 15	C 55 / 45 / 25	B 55 / 45 / 34	A 55 / 45 / 29	C 55 / 45 / 25	B 55 / 45 / 25	NS
9. Purdue Pegboard	50% / 34	A <10% / 23	Y	A <10% / 22	A 20% / 30	A 12% / 28	A 40% / 26	A 20% / 30	A <10% / 25	A 30% / 31	NS
10. Development Test of Visual-Motor Integration school 3/83	21-22 / 50%	A 15 / 4%	Y	A 15 / 4%	A 15 / 5%	A 17 / <5%	A 17 / <5%	A 17 / <5%	A 17 / <5%	A 17 / <5%	NS

Name **BRIAN W. (#2)** Age **13** years **5** months Sex **M** Drug **RITALIN** Dose **25 Mg** in his scores, they were definitely not in the direction of improvement.

On the Purdue Pegboard Brian initially exhibited a deficit. And this deficit persisted throughout the practice trials. No improvement appeared to take place as a result of medication and this was confirmed by the analysis of the data obtained from the 6 drug-assessment trials. On the Developmental Test of Visual-Motor Integration Brian also exhibited an initial deficit, and this deficit persisted throughout the practice trials. Analysis of the data obtained during the 6 drug-assessment trials revealed no evidence for improvement while on medication.

We can conclude from Brian W's data that tests #1–#5 and #8–#10 are not Ritalin sensitive. Although Brian's Steadiness Tester scores suggest the possibility of Ritalin sensitivity the p value of .10 does not lend great support to this possibility.

My final conclusion regarding Brian's scores on the PMAB is that none of the tests showed evidence for Ritalin sensitivity, with the exception of the Steadiness Tester with which the results are only mildly suggestive.

Roger M. (Patient #3)

Roger was first seen at age 11½ because of emotional immaturity, impulsivity, poor socialization, distractibility, hyperactivity (especially in the classroom), and impaired academic curiosity and motivation.

Roger's birth weight was 3 lbs. 8 oz. and he was considered to be small for gestational age (SGA). He spent 18 days in an incubator and was discharged from the hospital after 21 days. Although developmental milestones were normal, his coordination was described as always having been poor. Following a series of febrile convulsions at age 4 he continued to have occasional seizures, which were controlled with anticonvulsant medication.

As can be seen from Table 4-3 Roger's initial score on The Word Span Test was low, but improved to above average levels during the practice trials. Test scores during the 6 drug-assessment trials showed no significant differences between drug-free and post-drug scores. No impairments were seen in the next 3 tests of auditory attention (tests #2–#4); however, these instruments were still assessed to ascertain whether they were Ritalin sensitive. As can be seen from Table 4-3, there was no evidence that the 3 instruments were Ritalin sensitive.

Clinically, it was found that 25 mg. was the optimum dose for Roger. And this was verified by his improvement on the Steadiness Tester after Ritalin administration at that dosage level. Roger's initial score on the Steadiness Tester was abnormal and continued to be so during the first 4 of 5 practice trials. The scores obtained during the 6 drug-assessment trials did not indicate that the Steadiness Tester was Ritalin sensitive for Roger.

Roger's score on test #6 was normal but, because this is a test of visual attention, further trials, both practice and drug-assessment, were administered. Again, there was no evidence of Ritalin sensitivity, either for Roger's error score or the time it took him to complete the task. Tests #7 and #8 were normal and Ritalin sensitivity was not tested. The reader may have wondered by this point what criteria I utilized to decide whether or not to continue with practice and drug-assessment trials after a normal score has been initially obtained. The main critera were time and expense. In situations when these two considerations are not operative, I generally complete the full battery. Because these were factors for most patients, I focused primarily on those instruments in which an initial deficit was found. In addition, the further I got into the study, and the clearer it became that most of the instruments were showing no evidence for sensitivity to psychostimulant medication, I became less motivated to administer prac-

Table 4-3 Psychostimulant Medication Assessment Battery Tabulation of Data

Assessment Instrument	Norm.	Score	Defic.	Post-drug	Practice Trials	1 Drug free	2 Post drug	3 Drug free	4 Post drug	5 Drug free	6 Post drug	p
1. Word Span	34.5	A 23	Y	33	A 46 / A 42	A 48	C 67	B 20	A 61	C 33	B 29	
2. Compliance with Serial Verbal Instructions	18.9	A 15	N	15	A 22 / A 22	A 26	C 26	B 26	A 30	C 26	B 30	
3. Digit Span Digits Forward (WISC-R)	7.0	A 8	N	10	A 7 / A 8	A 10	C 11	B 9	A 9	C 9	B 10	
4. Digit Span Digits Backward (WISC-R)	4.9	A 6	N	8	A 5 / A 5	A 9	C 7	B 8	A 5	C 7	B 7	
5. Steadiness Tester	4.0	A 20.1	Y	6.9	A 15.73 / A 14.68, 24.52, 18.40, 4.01	A 43.82	A 4.60	A 6.91	A 7.30	A 4.02	A 3.61	
6. Cancellation of Rapidly Recurring Target Figures	3±3E 70±25"	A 0E 100"	N N	65" 29	A 0 65" / A 0 71"	A 71"	C 0 58"	B 0 59"	A 57"	C 0 70"	A 67"	
7. Reversals Frequency Test, Recognition	2.8	A 0	N		A	A	A	A	A	A	A	
8. Block Design (WISC-R)	RS-37 SS-11	A RS-32 SS-10	N		A	A	C	B	A	C	B	
9. Purdue Pegboard	50% 31	A <10% 21	Y	35% 29	A 55% 30 / A <10 24	A <10% 24	A 63% 33	A 57% 30	A 58% 32	A 63% 33	A 30% 27	
10. Development Test of Visual-Motor Integration	56%	A 43%	N		A	A	A	A	A	A	A	

Name Roger H (#3) Age 11 years 10 months 12 Sex M Drug Ritalin Dose 25mg tice and drug-assessment trials after normal scores were obtained. It was becoming apparent that most of the instruments (with the exception of the Steadiness Tester) were not showing drug sensitivity and the chances of their ultimately doing so became progressively smaller with each demonstration of nonsensitivity.

Roger's initial score on the Purdue Pegboard was low and this was consistent with the clinical history of poor coordination. However, his score was average in one of the practice trials and below the 10th percentile in another. His scores in the 6 drug-assessment trials did not reveal Ritalin sensitivity for this instrument. Last, Roger's score on test #10 was normal and no further Ritalin assessment was done.

My final conclusion regarding the administration of the PMAB to Roger was that none of the instruments proved to be Ritalin sensitive.

James T. (Patient #4)

James was referred at the age of 5½ by his school because of disruptive behavior in the classroom, poor attention, hyperactivity, and significant problems in his relationships with peers. These difficulties exhibited themselves at home as well. When younger, his father had significant difficulty learning how to read and, even as an adult, considered himself to be dyslexic.

As can be seen on Table 4-4, James' initial score on The Word Span Test was just within the low end of the normal range. One practice trial was below normal and the other again at the lower end of the normal range. Throughout most of the study utilizing the PMAB 5 mg. of Ritalin was used. However, toward the end 7.5 mg. twice a day was found to be more efficacious. As can be seen, James's scores during the first 4 drug-assessment trials were not affected by 5 mg. of Ritalin, but there was a slight improvement on 7.5 mg. Read-

Table 4-4 Psychostimulant Medication Assessment Battery Tabulation of Data

Assessment Instrument	Norm.	Score	Defic.	Practice Trials	1 Drug free	2 Post drug	3 Drug free	4 Post drug	5 Drug free	6 Post drug	p
1. Word Span	22.1	A 15	N	A 12 · A 15	A 15	C 15	B 15	A 14	C 12 ⃝	B 19 ⃝	NS
2. Compliance with Serial Verbal Instructions	12.7	A 7	Y	A 9 · A 9	A 9	C 5	B 7	A 5	C 5 ⃝	B 12 ⃝	NS
3. Digit Span Digits Forward (WISC-R)	4	A 2	Y	A 2 · A 2	A 2	C 3	B 3	A 4	C 2	B 2	NS
4. Digit Span Digits Backward (WISC-R)	1.6	A 2	N	A 0 · A 2	A 2	C 3	B 2	A 2	C 3	B 2	NS
5. Steadiness Tester	39	A 82	Y	A 100.1 · A 119.5	A 121.6	A 65.2	A 60.5	A 35.7	A 26.7 ⃝	A 20.7	
6. Cancellation of Rapidly Recurring Target Figures	13±4 / —	A 27 / 1	Y	A 27 · A 2*	A	C	B	A	C	B 26.6 / 12.2 ⃝ ← 7.5mg	<.001
7. Reversals Frequency Test, Recognition	24±11	A 40	Y	A 19 · A 38	A 40	A 43	A — DISCONTINUED	A	A	A	
8. Block Design (WISC-R) — Too Young		A		A	A	C	B	A	C	B	
9. Purdue Pegboard	15.5	A 14	N	A	A	A	A	A	A	A	
10. Development Test of Visual-Motor Integration	10	A 10.5	N	A	A	A	A	A	A	A	

Name James T. (#4)   Age 5 years 6+ months   Sex M   Drug Ritalin   Dose 5mg

ers who have had personal experience administering psycho-stimulant medication will verify its unpredictability. We know that, under the same conditions, there can be different rates of absorption of the medication into the bloodstream and even the total amount of medication absorbed into the bloodstream may differ on different days under seemingly similar or identical circumstances. In addition, many patients will lose sensitivity at a given dose level, but will regain it at a higher level. Again, the causes of these changes are often unknown. And this is what occurred in James' case. The net result, however, was no significant Ritalin sensitivity. On test #2 James revealed initial evidence for impairment, but this improvement did not exhibit itself during the practice trials during which his scores came within the low average range. In the first 4 of the 6 drug-assessment trials James was given 5 mg. of Ritalin and this dosage did not indicate any effect. When the dose was raised to 7.5 mg., improvement was noted but not enough to produce significant evidence that the instrument was Ritalin sensitive.

James's initial score on Test #3 showed evidence of impairment, an impairment that persisted through the practice trials. However, his scores during the 6 drug-assessment trials revealed no evidence that this instrument was Ritalin sensitive.

On test #4 an impairment was not found to be present. However, the 6 drug-assessment trials were administered and showed no evidence that this instrument is sensitive to Ritalin.

As mentioned, 5 mg. of Ritalin produced clinical change which seems to have been "lost" near the end of the period during which the PMAB was being administered. Accordingly, the dose was then raised to 7.5 mg. As seen on Table 4-4 James' initial score on the Steadiness Tester was abnormal and continued to be so during the practice trials. James's scores in the first 4 drug-assessment trials suggest that this instrument is Ritalin sensitive at the 5 mg. level. His scores in trials 5 and 6 also suggest Ritalin sensitivity at the 7.5 mg. dosage level. Analysis of the data indicated that these changes were significant at the p < .001 level.

It is very difficult to utilize The Reversals Frequency Test (#7) for children at the kindergarden level. Because they are just learning their letters, data regarding reversals frequency becomes difficult to assess. This problem can be partially circumvented by counting unknown errors at this age level. (R.A. Gardner, 1978). The average 5½ year old makes 24 ± 11 reversals errors. James' initial score was 40 errors and his 2 follow-up practice scores were 19 and 38 errors. There is a strong suggestion here that James was still in that category of children whose knowledge of letters was so meager that meaningful assessment of reversals was impractical and somewhat meaningless. The first 2 drug-assessment trial scores were 40 and 43 errors. At that point, I came to the conclusion that assessment of reversals frequency was meaningless for James and so further drug-assessment trials were not administered. James' initial scores on tests #9 and #10 were normal and therefore drug assessment trials were not administered.

My final conclusion with regard to James' PMAB assessment was that the only instrument that proved to be Ritalin sensitive was the Steadiness Tester.

Sean O. (Patient #5)

This 8-year-old boy was referred because of disruptive behavior in the classroom, hyperactivity, temper outbursts in response to minor frustrations, and poor commitment to his academic program. The parents were religious Catholics and strongly committed to a parochial school education. They recognized that the school he was attending was much more stringent than their local public school (both with regard to academic requirements and tolerance for atypical behavior) but, because of their deep religious convictions, the question of transfer to a more relaxed public school atmosphere was out of the question for them. Sean had gross and fine motor coordination problems, resulting in his doing very poorly in sports and this interfered with his socialization. No specific etiological factor for his symptoms could be found.

Both clinically and with the Steadiness Tester it was determined that the 10 mg. dose of Ritalin was optimum for him. As can be seen from Table 4-5, Sean's scores on the first 4 tests (which assess primarily auditory attention) were normal and so no further practice or drug-assessment trials were eliminated. However, he was given one post-drug assessment on each of these 4 tests (see column #6 under the Drug Assessment Trials) and, as can be seen, there was no suggestion of drug improvement with any of these 4 instruments.

Sean's score on the Steadiness Tester was definitely in the abnormal range and he persisted with high scores through the practice trials. As can be seen, there was marked improvement in each post-drug trial when compared to the previous drug-free trial, and these differences were statistically significant at the < .01 level.

On test #6, Sean's initial error score was in the normal range but his time score was abnormal. And this abnormality persisted through the practice trials. However, in the 6 drug-assessment trials he continued to exhibit problems in finishing the task in a short enough time to qualify being placed in the average range. There was no evidence that Ritalin improved his visual concentration here.

On test #7 Sean's initial score was in the normal range. Further practice trials were not administered nor the full series of drug-assessment trials. However, one further assessment was administered under post-drug conditions (see column #6 under Drug Assessment Trials) and there was no

Table 4-5 Psychostimulant Medication Assessment Battery Tabulation of Data

Assessment Instrument	Norm.	Score	Defic.	Practice Trials	Drug Assessment Trials						
					1 Drug free	2 Post drug	3 Drug free	4 Post drug	5 Drug free	6 Post drug	p
1. Word Span	28.7	A 37	N	A	A	C	B	A	C	B 37	
2. Compliance with Serial Verbal Instructions	17.0	A 18	N	A	A	C	B	A	C	B 16	
3. Digit Span Digits Forward (WISC-R)	5.8	A 7	N	A	A	C	B	A	C	B 7	
4. Digit Span Digits Backward (WISC-R)	3.7	A 3	N	A	A	C	B	A	C	B 2	
5. Steadiness Tester	8.2	A 53.4	Y	A 72.3 / A 61.6	A 98.1	A 17.2	A 80.3	A 26.8	A 126.2	A 49.0	<.01
6. Cancellation of Rapidly Recurring Target Figures	2±2 / 116±33"	A 2 / 260"	2 / Y	A 4 / 278" / 21	A – / 205" / 20	C 0 / 204"	B – / 242"	A – / 186"	C – / 172"	B 0 / 203"	NS
7. Reversals Frequency Test, Recognition	3.7	A 4	N	A	A	A	A	A	A	A 3	
8. Block Design (WISC-R)	55 / 10	A 55 / 12	N	A	A	C	B	A	C	B	
9. Purdue Pegboard	50% / 23	A <10% / 19	Y	A 30% / 21	A 10% / 19	A 78% / 26	A 78% / 26	A 78% / 26	A 78% / 26	A 75% / 28	NS
10. Development Test of Visual-Motor Integration	50% / 9.5	A 96% / 14.5	N	A	A	A	A	A	A	A	

Name __Scan O (#5)__   Age __8__ years __4__ months   Sex __M__   Drug __Ritalin__   Dose __10 mg__ evidence for improvement. In fact, his score was slightly lower.

Sean's initial scores on test #8 were above average. Accordingly, no practice trials nor drug-assessment trials were administered.Consistent with the clinical description of poor coordination, Sean's scores on test #9 were found to be below average. There was some improvement during the practice trials and even more improvement over the course of the drug-assessment trials. Analysis of these revealed no evidence that this test is Ritalin sensitive. Furthermore, there is good reason to believe that the practice effect played a role in his improvement and so might have beclouded any Ritalin sensitivity that might have been present.

On test #10 Sean's scores were significantly above average (96th percentile). Accordingly, no practice trials or drug-assessment trials were administered.

My conclusion is that Sean's visual attention was not improved by Ritalin and that the clinical observation that his hyperactivity was reduced by Ritalin was substantiated by his performance on the Steadiness Tester. Sean's case supports well the argument that Ritalin's effect is primarily at the motor level rather than at the attention-sustaining level.

David G. (Patient #6)

This 9½-year-old boy was referred because of hyperactivity, poor attention span, difficulty finishing his work in school, and impulsivity. He was of average intelligence and was functioning at grade level in reading, spelling, and arithmetic. His developmental milestones were in the average range as was his coordination. Clinically, Ritalin was not found to improve his behavior; however, Dexedrine 5 mg. twice a day did produce improvement.

As can be seen from Table 4-6 David's initial score on test #1 showed evidences for deficiency, which was maintained

Table 4-6 Psychostimulant Medication Assessment Battery Tabulation of Data

Assessment Instrument	Norm.	Score	Defic.	Practice Trials		Drug Assessment Trials						p
						1 Drug free	2 Post drug	3 Drug free	4 Post drug	5 Drug free	6 Post drug	
1. Word Span	33.3	A 23	Y	A 18Y	A 22Y	A 32N	C 32N	B 27	A 28	C 37	B 24	NS
2. Compliance with Serial Verbal Instructions	17.3	A 18	N	A	A	A	C	B	A	C	B	
3. Digit Span Digits Forward (WISC-R)	6.1	A 8	N	A	A	A	C	B	A	C	B	
4. Digit Span Digits Backward (WISC-R)	4.8	A 3	?N	A 24	A 5N	A 4N	C 4N	B 4	A 5	C 6	B 5	NS
5. Steadiness Tester	10.4	A 55.6	Y	A 52.6	A 61.6	A 82.5	A 35.6	A 31.5	A 24.0	A 28.0	A 21.7	NS
6. Cancellation of Rapidly Recurring Target Figures	3±3 20±24	A 7 86	Y?	A	A	A	C	B	A	C	B	
7. Reversals Frequency Test, Recognition	3.1	A 10	Y	A 11Y	A 10Y	A 13	A 3	A 2	A 6	A 11	A 3	NS
8. Block Design (WISC-R)	RS 22-25 55-10	A RS 19 55-9	N	A		A	C	B	A	C	B	
9. Purdue Pegboard	50% 56% 50% 50%	A <10 <10 <10	Y	A		A	A	A	A	A	A	
10. Development Test of Visual-Motor Integration	- 50% 16.5	A 19% 13.5	Y	A 12Y 12.5		A 35% 15.5	A 33% 16	A 15% 13	A 35% 15.5	A 48% 17	A 48% 17	NS

Name David G. (#6)   Age 9 years 10 months   Sex M   Drug Dexedrine   Dose 5mg during the practice trials. However, there was no evidence from analysis of the data obtained from the 6 drug-assessment trials that Dexedrine produced any improvement in his scores. His scores on tests #2 and #3 were in the normal range. Accordingly, no practice trials or drug-assessment trials were administered.

On test #4 David's score was in the low end of the average range. Accordingly, practice trials and drug-assessment trials were administered. His score on the 3rd practice trial and all 6 drug-assessment trials were average to above average and there was no evidence that this test was sensitive to Dexedrine.

David's score on the Steadiness Tester was definitely abnormal as were his scores during the 2 subsequent practice trials. During administration of the drug-assessment trials there appeared to be improvement following the administration of Dexedrine because each of the 3 post-drug scores was lower than his scores during each previous drug-free trial. However, the improvements were not great enough to be statistically significant.

On test #6 David's error score was slightly deficient but his time score was in the normal range. The decision was made not to give further practice and drug-assessment trials on this test, primarily because of time limitations.

David's score on test #7 was in the deficient realm and this deficiency persisted through the 2 practice trials. However, no significant improvement was noted over the course of the 6 drug- assessment trials.

On test #8 David's score was in the normal range. No practice and drug-assessment trials were administered. On test #9 David's scores were at the 10th percentile and below. No further testing, either practice trials or drug assessment trials was done.

On test #10 a mild deficit was found to be present, both in the initial testing and the one practice trial. David's scores during the drug-assessment trials showed no evidence that Dexedrine was improving his performance on this task.

My final conclusion with regard to David's scores on the PMAB was that none of the 10 tests were Dexedrine sensitive, although the Steadiness Tester showed suggestive promise for such sensitivity.

Norman L. (Patient #7)

This 10-year-old boy was referred because of angry acting out in school and provocation of his teachers and principal. His general attitude was that of a wise-guy and smart-aleck. He was disruptive in the classroom, exhibited poor concentration, was impulsive and showed diminished commitment to his academic pursuits. Accordingly, there was a steady deterioration of his grades. He was of average intelligence and there was no evidence for a neurologically based learning disability. There was no improvement on 10 mg. Ritalin twice a day, but there was on 20 mg. twice a day, in that he became more compliant in the classroom and less active.

Norman's scores were in the normal range on all 4 tests of auditory attention (#1–#4). Because his initial score on test was just within the normal range, the decision was made to administer the practice trials as well as the 6 drug-assessment trials. As can be seen from the Table 4-7, of the 6 drug-assessment trials there was improvement in each drug-free/post-drug set following the administration of Ritalin – an improvement which was significant at the < .05 level. No further practice trials or drug-assessment trials were administered for Tests #2–#4.

On test #5 the score, although elevated, was still less than one standard deviation above the mean (+0.82 s.d.). Norman's scores on the 2 subsequent practice trials were, however, more than one standard deviation above the mean. As can be seen from his scores over the 6 drug-assessment trials, there was improvement in each drug-free/post-drug set

Table 4-7 Psychostimulant Medication Assessment Battery Tabulation of Data

Assessment Instrument	Norm.	Score	Defic.	Practice Trials		Drug Assessment Trials							A
						1 Drug free	2 Post drug	3 Drug free	4 Post drug	5 Drug free	6 Post drug	p	
1. Word Span	33.4	A 27	N	A 27	A 37	A 32	C 39	B 33	A 38	C 33	B 37	<.05	.352
2. Compliance with Serial Verbal Instructions	20.0	A 18	N	A	A	A	C	B	A	C	B		
3. Digit Span Digits Forward (WISC-R)	5.9	A 5	N	A	A	A	C	B	A	C	B		
4. Digit Span Digits Backward (WISC-R)	4.3	A 4	N	A	A	A	C	B	A	C	B		
5. Steadiness Tester	8.8	A 14.8	N	A 16.3	A 21.7	A 36.3	A 5.0	A 25.3	A 8.9	A 34.3	A 4.3	<.05	.359
6. Cancellation of Rapidly Recurring Target Figures	3±3	A 5	N	A	A	A	C	B	A	C	B		
7. Reversals Frequency Test, Recognition	2	A 1	<N	A	A	A	A	A	A	A	A		
8. Block Design (WISC-R)	50% RS-10	A 25% RS-8	<N	A	A	A	C	B	A	C	B		
9. Purdue Pegboard	26.3	A 23	<N	A	A	A	A	A	A	A	A		
10. Development Test of Visual-Motor Integration	50% RS-19	A 68% RS-19		A	A	A	A	A	A	A	A		

Name NORMAN L (#7)   Age 10 years 0 months   Sex M   Drug Ritalin   Dose 20 mg after the administration of Ritalin. This improvement was found to be significant at the p < .05 level.

Norman's scores on tests #6–#10 were basically within the normal range and further testing was not administered.

My final conclusion with regard to Norman's scores were that tests #1 and #5 demonstrated suggestive evidence of being sensitive to Ritalin.

Larry R. (Patient #8)

Larry, a 10½-year-old boy, was in a special class for children with neurologically based learning disabilities. His IQ was in the low to mid-80s. He also exhibited impulsivity, distractability, hyperactivity, and inappropriate laughing. He was referred because Ritalin, Cylert, Mellaril, and Haldol had not proven effective in improving his behavior. Accordingly, I chose to assess the effects of Dexedrine on his behavior and to include him in the PMAB study.

As can be seen from Table 4-8 Larry exhibited deficiencies on 9 of the 10 tests of the PMAB. In addition, his impairments were sometimes moderate to severe (many below the 10th percentile).

All 4 tests of auditory attention (#1–#4) showed deficits that persisted through the practice trials. In addition, on all 4 tests there was no evidence that Dexedrine improved performance; accordingly, there was no evidence that any of these 4 instruments was Dexedrine sensitive.

Larry's deficiencies on test #5 persisted through the practice trials. As can be seen from the data obtained during the drug-assessment trials, there was improvement in each of the 3 drug free/post drug sets following the administration of Dexedrine. This improvement was significant at the p < .05 level.

On test #6 Larry exhibited impairments both with regard to his error score as well as the time it took him to complete the

Table 4-8 Psychostimulant Medication Assessment Battery Tabulation of Data

Assessment Instrument	Norm.	Score	Defic.	Practice Trials	Drug Assessment Trials						p
					1 Drug free	2 Post drug	3 Drug free	4 Post drug	5 Drug free	6 Post drug	
1. Word Span	33.9	A 12	Y	A 15	A 15	C 12	B 12	A 15	C 12	B 19	NS
2. Compliance with Serial Verbal Instructions	19.3	A 9	Y	A 12	A 9	C 12	B 12	A 9	C 9	B 10	NS
3. Digit Span Digits Forward (WISC-R)	7.2	A 2	Y	A 3	A 2	C 2	B 4	A 3	C 2	B 2	NS
4. Digit Span Digits Backward (WISC-R)	5.0	A 2	Y	A 3	A 2	C 3	B 2	A 2	C 3	B 3	NS
5. Steadiness Tester	8.8	A 29.0	Y	A 79.6 71.7	A 22.8	C 44	B 42.1	A 6.6	C 47.9	A 6.7	<.05
6. Cancellation of Rapidly Recurring Target Figures	2±2E 90"±24"	5E 134"	Y Y	7E 62" A 12E 87"	0E 203"	C 1E 169"	B 4wE 57"	A 8E 95"	C 0E 225"	B 0E 205"	NS NS
7. Reversals Frequency Test, Recognition	2.0	3	N	A	A	A	A	A	A	A	
8. Block Design (WISC-R)	RS 26-30 SS 10	RS 1-5 6	Y	A RS-19 SS-8	A RS-17 SS-7	C RS-15 SS-7	B RS-19 SS-8	A RS-20 SS-8	C RS-14 SS-6	B RS-26 SS-10	NS
9. Purdue Pegboard	RS-28 50%	RS-18 <10%	Y	A RS-24 RS-18 35% <10%	A RS-26 35%	C RS-30 RS-25 60-70% 35%	B RS-26 35%	A RS-25 RS-13 25% 5%	C RS-25 RS-13 25% 5%	A RS-32 85%	NS
10. Development Test of Visual-Motor Integration	RS-19 50%	A RS-4 4%	Y	A RS-10 RS-9 <5% 4%	A RS-11 <5%	A RS-15 5+%	A RS-10 <5%	A RS-13 5+%	A RS-13 5+%	A RS-15 5+%	<.05

Name **LARRY R (#8)**   Age **10** years **8** months   Sex **M**   Drug **Dexedrine**   Dose **.75 mg** task. The error deficit persisted through the practice trials; whereas the time deficit did not, suggesting improvement by practice effect. The figures obtained during the drug-assessment trials revealed no evidence for improvement with Dexedrine. The reader should note that Larry made 46 errors on one administration during the drug-free state (column #3). It was during this administration that he took only 57 seconds (his fastest time)—suggesting that he was racing through the test and not attending properly to the task.

On test #8 Larry's initial score was deficient and his deficiency persisted through the practice trials. As can be seen from the scores obtained during the drug-assessment trials, there was no evidence of improvement on Dexedrine, nor that this instrument is Dexedrine sensitive.

On test #9 Larry's score was initially deficient and it was also deficient on one of the 2 practice trials. His scores, however, were not deficient throughout all 6 drug-assessment trials, nor was there evidence that there was any improvement as a result of the Dexedrine. As mentioned, I believe that the practice effect operates strongly in the improvement one sees on this instrument—making it difficult thereby to assess the effects of psychostimulant medication.

On test #10 Larry exhibited a significant deficiency that persisted throughout the practice trials. An evaluation of the drug-assessment trials indicates improvement in the post-drug phase in all three drug-free/post-drug sets. This improvement was significant at the $p < .05$ level.

My final conclusion with regard to Larry's PMAB was that test #5 and test #10 were the only ones that appeared to be sensitive to Dexedrine, but at the $p < .05$ level, not an impressive level of significance.

Alvin C. (Patient # 9)

This 9½-year-old boy was referred because of hyperactive and impulsive behavior in the classroom. In addition he was antisocial, both in school and at home. He was an extremely bright boy and his IQ on the WISC-R was at the 99th percentile level. There were many factors throughout the pregnancy, however, that placed Alvin at high risk for the development of organic brain dysfunction. His mother smoked on the average of 1 package of cigarettes a day. His mother hemorrhaged large clots during the pregnancy in association with placenta previa and transverse positioning of the fetus. Accordingly, he was delivered by Caesarean section. His birth weight was 4 lbs. 11 oz. and he was considered small for gestational age (SGA).

As can be seen from Table 4-9 Alvin's scores were in the normal range on all 10 tests of the PMAB. Although his initial score on test #5 was high (consistent with the clinical observation of hyperactivity) it was within 1 standard deviation of the mean. His 1 practice trial was also elevated. As can be seen from the drug-assessment trial scores, there was no evidence that Ritalin was improving his scores. As is obvious, it is much more difficult to establish that Ritalin reduces hyperactivity when the Steadiness Tester scores are initially in the normal range. In such cases, one must question whether the child is indeed hyperactive. The child could be hyperactive in the clinical situation, but the Steadiness Tester is not reflecting the clinical hyperactivity. Whatever the reasons, when the Steadiness Tester scores are in the normal range one is not likely to be able to ascertain this instrument's sensitivity to psychostimulant medication.

Reasons for Discontinuing the Study After Assessing Nine Patients

Some readers may have wondered why I have seen fit to publish data with only 9 patients. As I am sure the reader can appreciate, the administration of the PMAB is quite time consuming. The administration of all 10 tests generally takes

Table 4-9 Psychostimulant Medication Assessment Battery Tabulation of Data

Assessment Instrument	Norm.	Score	Defic.	Practice Trials	1 Drug free	2 Post drug	3 Drug free	4 Post drug	5 Drug free	6 Post drug	p
1. Word Span	30.6	A 37	N	A	A	C	B	A	C	B	
2. Compliance with Serial Verbal Instructions	16.5	A 18	N	A	A	C	B	A	C	B	
3. Digit Span Digits Forward (WISC-R)	6.2	A 7	N	A	A	C	B	A	C	B	
4. Digit Span Digits Backward (WISC-R)	4.3	A 7	N	A	A	C	B	A	C	B	
5. Steadiness Tester	10.4	A 16.8	N	A 20.3	A 7.3	A 8.6	A 14.1	A 10.5	A 15.7	A 12.8	NS
6. Cancellation of Rapidly Recurring Target Figures	2±2 116	A 0ᵉ 105	N	A	A	C	B	A	C	B	
7. Reversals Frequency Test, Recognition	3	A 2	N	A	A	A	A	A	A	A	
8. Block Design (WISC-R)	55-10 55-17 85 RS-21-24 46	A	N	A	A	C	B	A	C	B	
9. Purdue Pegboard	24+4	A 34	N	A	A	A	A	A	A	A	
10. Development Test of Visual-Motor Integration	15	A 19.5 85%	N	A	A	A	A	A	A	A	

Name Alvin C. (#9)   Age 9 years 5 months   Sex M   Drug Ritalin   Dose 10mg between 1 and 2 hours, depending upon the child's speed and cooperation. These factors, however, should not have been the primary ones for determing whether or not further testing with more patients was justified. The main reason for not continuing the testing was that there was not enough evidence on the basis of the first 9 patients to give me any hope that any of the tests (other than #5) would prove useful as an instrument for monitoring psychostimulant medication. In order for one of the other 9 tests to ultimately prove useful for this purpose I would have to have hundreds who would demonstrate such sensitivity in order to counterbalance the original findings of nonsensitivity. I would have had to believe that I had extremely bad luck in my patient selection and that there is a large sea of children out there who indeed would demonstrate such sensitivity, but unfortunately I had not tapped this source. Not believing this to be likely, I decided to conclude the study with the 9 patients. Accordingly, I am back to using the Steadiness Tester as my monitoring instrument for psychostimulant medication. I am still, however, thinking about the problem and hope that another instrument may come my way that may lend itself to such utilization. If and when that time comes, I will once again utilize the PMAB for the purpose of assessing this instrument and hope that there may be readers who will similarly utilize it for this purpose.

The Continuous Performance Test (CPT)

Some readers may have wondered why I did not include the *Continuous Performance Test (CPT)* in the battery, especially because it has been described as being useful for assessing objectively the effects of psychostimulant medication on concentration. In the visual form of the test, a stream of randomized letters is flashed before the child at the rate of one every 1 to 2 seconds. In a typical task the child is instructed to press a button every time an X appears which has been preceded by an A. The child is told *not* to press the button when an X is preceded by any other letter or when an A is preceded by an X. (Of course any other combination of letters could be used.) The target sequences appear aperiodically. An auditory modification of the test is also used in which the child hears rather than views the letter sequences. The test requires sustained concentration and is very sensitive to deficiencies in this area. The greater the number of errors the more poorly the child is considered to be concentrating. However, impulsive children are also likely to make more errors than normal because they press the button too quickly, rather than waiting long enough to be sure that the proper combination of letters has indeed appeared. Another measurement that may be taken on the CPT is reaction time. Again, the impulsive child is more likely to have a short reaction time. Last, impaired concentration on a psychogenic basis is also going to result in an abnormally high number of errors on the CPT, and this is an important consideration when evaluating the meaning of a child's poor performance.

V.I. Douglas (1972 and 1974) compared normal and hyperactive children's scores on the CPT for both visual and auditory stimuli (using the X preceded by an A stimulus sequence). She found that hyperactive children made significantly more errors, made more impulsive responses, and deteriorated more rapidly than normals. She considered the attentional deficit and impulsivity to explain the hyperactive children's impaired performance. D. Sykes et al. (1972), using the same X followed by an A target sequence, similarly found that hyperactive children made more incorrect responses and fewer correct responses than normals.

Unfortunately, CPT equipment is extremely expensive (about $8,000 a unit) and so has never enjoyed widespread popularity, even among laboratory workers. Because of its cost, 25 times more than the Steadiness Tester, I myself do not own a unit and so did not consider it in this study—especially because the primary purpose of the study was to find an inexpensive test for monitoring psychostimulant medication. I do not doubt that the CPT is sensitive to psychostimulant medication and that it can be used to monitor such drugs. However, on the basis of my findings here, I suspect that the improvement on this task that one obtains after the administration of psychostimulant medication is *more related to the motor element than the attentional*. The child is asked to press a button (a motor task) and it has been demonstrated by J.L. Rapoport that Dexedrine shortens children's reaction times on this test (1978).

FINAL CONCLUSIONS

Table 4-10 provides a summary of the findings of all 9 patients presented. Of the 10 tests in the PMAB only one (the Steadiness Tester) showed suggestive evidence for sensitivity to psychostimulant medication and thereby showed promise for utilization as an instrument for monitoring such medication. On this point, then, I was back to where I had started prior to setting up the study. I consider myself to have been unsuccessful in finding a pencil-and-paper test that could be useful for monitoring psychostimulant medication. As can be seen from Table 4-10 there were suggestions at times that other tests (#1, #4 and #10) were sensitive to the effects of psychostimulant medication, but these examples were so isolated and the level of sensitivity so low ($p < .05$ and $p < .01$) that I was not able to conclude that these instruments were indeed sensitive to psychostimulant medication.

Hyperactivity

Test #5 showed confirmation of my previous clinical observations that the Steadiness Tester could prove useful as an

Table 4-10 Psychostimulant Medication Assessment Battery-Total Study p Values

Assessment Instrument	#1	#2	#3	#4	#5	#6	#7	#8	#9
					Patients				
1. Word Span	NS	NS	NS	NS		NS	<.05	NS	
2. Compliance with Serial Verbal Instructions	NS	NS	NS	NS				NS	
3. Digit Span Digits Forward (WISC-R)	NS (<.10)	NS	NS	NS		NS		NS	
4. Digit Span Digits Backward (WISC-R)	<.01	NS	NS	NS		NS		NS	
5. Steadiness Tester	<.001	NS (<0.10)	NS	<.001	<.01	NS	<.05	<.05	NS
6. Cancellation of Rapidly Recurring Target Figures	NS (<.10) NS	NS NS	NS NS		NS NS			NS NS	
7. Reversals Frequency Test, Recognition	NS					NS			
8. Block Design (WISC-R)	NS							NS	
9. Purdue Pegboard	NS	NS	NS		NS			NS	
10. Development Test of Visual-Motor Integration	NS					NS		<.05	

instrument for monitoring psychostimulant medication. Patients #1 and #4 exhibited extreme sensitivity (p < .001). It is of interest that one of these patients (#4) had the highest initial score of all 9 patients in the group and the other (#1) ranked 4th of the 9. This is consistent with my previous observation that the higher the patient's score on the Steadiness Tester the greater the likelihood it will be sensitive to psychostimulant medication. In contrast, the closer the child's initial scores are to the average the less the likelihood that the child's score on the instrument will be affected by psychostimulant medication. Three of the 9 patients (#3, #6, and #9) showed no evidence that Ritalin was helping their scores on the Steadiness Tester. This is consistent with my clinical observation that psychostimulant medication is not effective in reducing the activity levels of about 25 percent of children.

Whereas there was once a prevailing notion that psychostimulant medication could be used to differentiate between psychogenic and organic hyperactivity, most examiners in the field today agree that it makes no such differentiation. Earlier investigators went so far as to state that it was of diagnostic value and that if the child's hyperactivity was reduced by psychostimulant medication then it was thereby organic and if the hyperactivity was not reduced it had to be psychogenic. My own experience has been that Ritalin cannot differentiate between these two forms of hyperactivity and that it "doesn't care." At whatever level it may be acting, it blocks activity level. Accordingly, the reader does well not to concern him- or herself with whether a child's high activity level in this study was organic or psychogenic. As mentioned in Chapter One, I believe this to be a crucial consideration (often ignored in recent years); but it is *not* a consideration for this aspect of my study. One might think about whether my patients' hyperactivity was organic or psychogenic for other purposes. For the purposes of this study I was only concerned with whether the hyperactivity was reflecting itself with high scores on the Steadiness Tester and, if so, whether psycho-stimulant medication would be effective in improving scores on the Steadiness Tester—with the implication that such im-provement on this instrument would parallel clinical im-provement (confirming thereby my clinical observations).

Attention-Sustaining Capacity

I believe that one of the most important things to come out of this study was the surprising failure of tests #1, #4, and #6 to be Ritalin sensitive. There are thousands of articles in the liter-ature describing the effects of psychostimulant medication on attention. Many of these studies come to this conclusion on the basis of questionnaires and scales such as those of Connor (see Chapter Three). The jump is made between a score on a particular questionnaire and attentional capacity. It is of inter-est that before DSM-III was published in 1980, the same scales were used to assess for the presence of hyperactivity. Here, I have focussed specifically on instruments that assess objec-tively attention-sustaining capacity. There was no strong evi-dence for improvement on any of these instruments following the administration of psychostimulant medication. These findings shed doubt on the belief that psychostimulant medi-cation improves attention, or at least attention-sustaining ca-pacity as measured by these four instruments.

This finding is consistent with my clinical observations that children who have been diagnosed as having ADD do not generally show isolated deficits on those 3 subtests of the WISC-R that assess to a significant degree attention-sus-taining capacity: Arithmetic, Digit Span, and Coding. These findings lend substantiation to my belief that there is no such clinical entity as an attention deficit disorder. All of the chil-dren in this study were clinically hyperactive. That was the primary criterion for including them in the study. Some of these children did indeed have low scores on some of the au-ditory attention tests (#1–#4) and others did not. Many of those who did show evidence for attentional impairment also manifested impairments in other areas (tests #6–#10). There was *no* child who exhibited isolated impairments in Tests ✳ #1–#4 and no impairments at all in other areas. Such children, if they exist, would have to be considered to be suffering with ADD. Although only 9 patients are discussed in this study, and although all 9 were hyperactive, none of them exhibited isolated deficits in tests #1–#4 and no impairments in tests #6–#10. This also lends confirmation to my belief that an isolated attention-sustaining deficit, without any other signs or symptoms of neurological impairment, does not exist. ADD *as an isolated clinical entity* does exist in the minds of those who believe in its existence; but it does not exist if one takes the trouble to demonstrate its existence objectively.

Not only does my data lend support to my view that there is no such entity as an isolated impairment warranting the name ADD, but that even those children who do have attention-sustaining impairment are not likely to enjoy improvements of their attention by the administration of psychostimulant medication. If, however, they are hyperactive—definitely a separate entity—then they may *appear* to be paying attention better after the administration of psychostimulant medication. However, this improvement in their attention is not, I believe, the result of the affect of psychostimulant medication on attention-sustaining capacity; but rather on its capacity to reduce hyperactivity. This is another important finding of this study, namely, that psychostimulant medication reduces hyperactivity but does not improve attention. This lends confirmation to my view that hyperactivity and attention-sustaining deficits (if and when they exist) are two separate entities.

Compliance

Parents traditionally state that psychostimulant medication helps their children "pay attention better" or "listen better." I am in agreement that this is a common statement made by the mothers of these children. However, when one questions them further, one often learns that these children have no problem paying attention to television and will be "glued to the set" for hours at a time. If one inquires further about what the parents are talking about when they say that the child is "paying attention better," one finds that they are really talking about *compliance*. When they say that the child "listens better" they are talking again about compliance. The child will be described to be complying with requests and instructions in a more cooperative way. Test #2 was devised in the attempt to assess objectively this particular function. The study does not indicate that the instrument proved to be sensitive to psychostimulant medication. All 5 children who were administered the drug-assessment trials (patients #1, #2, #3, #4 and #8) showed no evidence for improvement on this instrument after the administration of psychostimulant medication. There are 2 possibilities here. One is that the aforementioned statement that psychostimulant medication improves compliance is incorrect or that the instrument itself is not adequately assessing this function. I believe the latter interpretation is the more likely one. The test is just not close enough to the situation at home where the child is being asked to do such things as dress, pick up clothing, take out the garbage, and perform other unpleasant tasks. In contrast, children often are strongly motivated to comply with the challenges of this test, which is somewhat reminiscent of the traditional childhood game *Simple Simon*. (Perhaps I should have devised a test which involved instructions relating to such tasks as taking out the garbage, picking up one's dirty socks, etc.)

Other Functions Assessed by the PMAB

There is also no evidence that tests #7–#10 were sensitive to psychostimulant medication. Accordingly, the results do not substantiate reports that psychostimulant medication reduces reversals frequency (#7), improves visual-perception (#8), reduces impaired fine motor coordination (#9), or improves visual-motor integration (#10).

Final Concluding Statement

My general clinical observations have led me to the conclusion that Ritalin does three things. First, it reduces hyperactivity. Second, it improves compliance. And third, it reduces impulsivity. This study did not focus on the impulsivity issue. Again, it is very difficult to devise an instrument that assesses specifically this function. The Mazes subtest of the WISC-R can be used for this purpose as can *The Matching Familiar Figures Test* (J. Kagan, 1964). The Mazes test does not lend itself well to utilization in the PMAB because of the improvement that quickly comes with practice. And Kagan's test does not fall into the category of a simple pencil-and-paper test. Nor could I find other pencil-and-paper tests that purport to assess for the presence of impulsivity. Accordingly, I hoped that at least one of the 10 tests I did finally select would prove useful for assessing objectively the effects of psychostimulant medication.

Whereas previously I was of the belief that Ritalin improves attention, I no longer hold this view. This study supports the position that psychostimulant medication reduces hyperactivity and does not improve attention. It sheds no light on the issue of whether psychostimulant medication improves compliance and/or reduces impulsivity. My hope is that my study will play a role in dispelling the myth of the existence of an isolated attention deficit disorder and that it will contribute to the appreciation of the importance of assessing objectively various signs and symptoms subsumed under the GMBDS rubric.

At the end of Chapter Two I commented on the implications of my theory for the diagnosis and treatment of children with attentional deficits. I believe that the data presented in these final 2 chapters lend support to my view that there is no such entity as an attention-deficit disorder. Most of the children so diagnosed, I believe, are suffering with a psychogenic disturbance which may have as a contributing factor the genetic high activity-assertiveness factor (necessary for hunters and warriors) that was important for survival in past centuries and which makes it difficult for some children to sit for 6 to 7 hours a day in a classroom.

The attractiveness of the ADD diagnosis is consistent with the recent trend in psychiatry to embrace biological explanations for a wide variety of phenomena that were viewed as psychogenic in the 1930s through the 1960s. Although biological psychiatry has certainly made its contributions, I believe that the pendulum has swung too far in the biological direction. Psychodynamic therapies are time-consuming and expensive. The factors that have contributed to such symptoms are complex and have often existed for generations. The biological explanation is not only attractive to patients, who want quick cures, but to therapists who don't have the patience for the more laborious psychotherapeutic routes to alleviation. The biological approach is certainly an attractive one. Rather than spend long periods going into background history; rather than undergo the tedious process of trying to understand the multiplicity of factors that have produced the symptoms; all one has to do is supply the medicine that presumably will correct the biological abnormality that is theorized to be the cause of the disorder.

When it comes to obtaining grants, biologically oriented psychiatrists are obviously at an advantage over those who want to investigate the longer and presumably less predictably successfull forms of treatment. These financial considerations have contributed to a dehumanization of psychiatric care. The biological approach is also more attractive to schools and institutions were large numbers of patients must be "processed" and provided services. There was a time when doctors treated patients. Now the lingo calls us "providers" and our treatment "delivery of services." The terms conjure up visions of our driving pick-up and delivery trucks. Those who fund such research and treatment are more likely to be attracted to these presumably more "cost-effective" forms of therapy. The result of all of this is that the "customer" is being ripped off. The "product" being provided is often of specious, if of any, value at all. And the ADD diagnosis and its treatment is an excellent example of this pehnomenon. My hope is that this book will play some role in not only reversing this trend but contribute as well to our understanding of the psychiatric disorders of childhood which I refer to as the Group of Minimal Brain Dysfunction Syndromes.

References

Apgar, V. (1953), A proposal for a new method of evaluation of the newborn infant. *Anesthesia and Anelgesia* 32:260.

_____Holaday, D.A., James, L.S., Weisbrot, I.M., and Berrien, C. (1958), Evaluation of the newborn infant: second report. *Journal of the American Medical Association*, 168:1985-1988.

Ayres, A.J. (1968), *Southern California Perceptual-Motor Tests*. Los Angeles: Western Psychological Services.

Beery, K.E. and Buktenica, N.A. (1982), *Developmental Test of Visual-Motor Integration*. Chicago: Follett Publishing Co.

Bell, R.Q., Waldrop, M.F., and Weller, G.M. (1972), A rating system for the assessment of hyperactive and withdrawn children in preschool samples. *American Journal of Orthopsychiatry*, 42:23-24.

Bender, L. (1938), *A Visual Motor Gestalt Test and Its Clinical Use*. Research Monograph No. 3. New York: American Orthopsychiatric Association.

_____(1946) *Bender Motor Gestalt Test: Cards and Manual of Instructions*. New York: American Orthopsychiatric Association.

_____(1947), Clinical Study of 100 schizophrenic children. *American Journal of Orthopsychiatry*, 17:40-56.

Bennett, G.K., Seashore, H.G., and Wesman, A.G. (1974), *Differential Aptitude Tests*. New York: The Psychological Corporation.

Benton, A.L. (1970), Neuropsychological aspects of mental retardation. *The Journal of Special Education*, 4:3-11.

Brain, W. and Wilkinson, M. (1959), Observations on the extensor plantar reflex and its relationship to the functions of the pyramidal tract. *Brain*, 82:297:320.

Brock, S. (1945), *The Basis of Clinical Neurology*. Baltimore: The Williams & Wilkins Co.

Burgemeister, B.B., Blum, L.H., and Lorge, I. (1972), *Columbia Mental Maturity Scale*. New York: Harcourt Brace Jovanovich, Inc.

Charlton, M. (1973), *Clinical Aspects of Minimal Brain Dysfunction*. (one hour cassette tape). Behavioral Sciences Tape Library. Teaneck, New Jersey: Sigma Information, Inc.

Conners, C.K. (1969), A teacher rating scale for use in drug studies with children. *American Journal of Psychiatry*, 126:884-888.

_____(1970), Symptom patterns in hyperkinetic, neurotic, and normal children. *Child Development*, 41:667-682.

_____(1973), Parents' Questionnaire. *Psychopharmacology Bulletin*, pp. 231-234. Department of Health, Education, and Welfare Publication No. (HSM) 73-9002. Washington, D.C.:U.S. Government Printing Office.

Davids, A. (1971), An objective instrument for assessing hyperkinesis in children. *Journal of Learning Disabilities*, 4:499-501.

de Hirsch, K. (1974), Early Language development. In: *American Handbook of Psychiatry*, ed. S. Arieti, 2nd edit., Vol. I., pp. 352-367. New York:Basic Books, Inc.

Diagnostic and Statistical Manual of the American Psychiatric Association (DSM-III) (1980). Washington, D.C.: American Psychiatric Association.

Douglas, V.I. (1972), Stop, look and listen:The problem of sustained attention and impulse control in hyperactive and normal children. Canadian Journal of Behavioral Science, 4:259:282.

_____(1974), Differences between normal and hyperkinetic children. In: *Clinical Use of Stimulant Drugs in Children*, ed. C.R. Conners, North Chicago, Illinois: Abbott Laboratories, pp.12-23.

Fisher, M. (1956), Left hemiplegia and motor impersistence. *Journal of Nervous and Mental Diseases*, 123:201-218.

Frostig, M. (1961), *Developmental Test of Visual Perception*. Palo Alto, California: Consulting Psychologists Press.

Gardner, R.A. (1969), The guilt reaction of parents of children with severe physical disease. *American Journal of Psychiatry*, 126:636-644.

_____(1973a), *MBD: The Family Book About Minimal Brain Dysfunction*. New York: Jason Aronson, Inc.

_____(1973b), Psychotherapy of the psychogenic problems secondary to minimal brain dysfunction. *International Journal of Child Psychotherapy*, 2:224-256.

_____(1974a), The mutual storytelling technique in the treatment of psychogenic problems secondary to minimal brain dysfunction. *Journal of Learning Disabilities*, 7:135-143.

_____(1974b), Psychotherapy of minimal brain dysfunction. In: *Current Psychiatric Therapies*, ed. J. Masserman, Vol. XIV, pp. 15-21, New York: Grune & Stratton.

_____(1975a), Techniques for involving the child with MBD in meaningful psychotherapy. *Journal of Learning Disabilities*, 8:16-26.

_____(1975b), Psychotherapy in minimal brain dysfunction. In: *Current Psychiatric Therapies*, ed. J. Masserman, Vol. XV, pp. 25-38, New York: Grune & Stratton.

_____(1975c), *Dr. Gardner Talks to Children with Minimal Brain Dysfunction* (one-hour cassette tape). Cresskill, New Jersey: Creative Therapeutics.

_____(1978), *The Reversals Frequency Test*. Cresskill, New Jersey: Creative Therapeutics.

_____(1979), *The Objective Diagnosis of Minimal Brain Dysfunction*. Cresskill, New Jersey: Creative Therapeutics.

_____ and Broman, M. (1979a), The Purdue Pegboard; normative data on 1334 school children. *Journal of Clinical Child Psychology*, 8(3):156:162.

_____ _____(1979b), Letter reversals frequency in normal and MBD children. *Journal of Clinical Child Psychology*, 8(3):146-152.

_____Gardner, A.K., Caemmerer, A., and Broman, M. (1979), An instrument for measuring hyperactivity and other signs of minimal brain dysfunction. *Journal of Clinical Child Psychology*, 8(3):173:179.

_____(1981), Digits forward and digits backward as two separate tests: Normative data on 1567 school children. *Journal of Clinical Child Psychology*, 10(2):131-135.

_____(1983a), The Word Span Test. (Unpublished)

_____(1983b), Compliance with Serial Verbal Instructions. (Unpublished)

_____(1986), *The Psychotherapeutic Techniques of Richard A. Gardner*. Cresskill, New Jersey: Creative Therapeutics.

_____(1987), *The Diagnosis and Treatment of Psychogenic Learning Disabilities*. Cresskill, New Jersey: Creative Therapeutics. (in press).

_____*Psychotherapy of the Psychogenic Problems of Children with Neurologically Based Learning Disabilities*. Cresskill, New Jersey: Creative Therapeutics. (in press)

Garfield, J.C., Benton, A.L., and MacQueen, J. (1966), Motor impersistence in brain-damaged children. *Neurology*, 14:434-440.

Geschwind, N. (1965a), Disconnexion syndromes in animals and man, Part I. *Brain*, 88:237-294.

_____(1965b), Disconnexion syndromes in animals and man, Part II, *Brain*, 88:585-644.

_____(1971), Aphasia. *New England Journal of Medicine*, 284(12): 654-656.

_____(1972), Language and the Brain. *Scientific American*, 226(4): 76-83.

Goldman, R., Fristoe, M., and Woodcock, W. (1974), *Auditory Selective Attention Test*. Circle Pines, Minnesota: American Guidance Service, Inc.

Ingram, T. (1973), Soft signs. *Developmental Medicine and Child Neurology*, 15:527-530.

Kagan, J. (1964) *The Matching Familiar Figures Test*. Cambridge, Massachusetts: Harvard University.

Kirk, S.A., McCarthy, J.J., and Kirk, W.D. (1968), *The Illinois Test of Psycholinguistic Abilities*, rev. edit. Urbana, Illinois: University of Illinois Press.

Klein, D.F. and Gittelman-Klein, R. (1974), Diagnosis of minimal brain dysfunction and hyperkinetic syndrome. In: *Clinical Use of Stimulant Drugs in Children*, ed. C.K. Conners. North Chicago, Illinois: Abbott Laboratories, pp. 1-11.

Owen, F.W., Adams, P.A., Forrest, T., Stolz, L.M., and Fisher, S. (1971), Learning disorders in children: sibling studies. *Monographs of the Society for Research in Child Development*, 36(4):1-75, Serial No. 144.

Paine, R. and Oppe, T. (1966), *Neurological Examination of Children*. Clinicsin Developmental Medicine, Vol. 20/21. Spastics International Medical Publications. London: William Heinemann Medical Books Ltd.; Philadelphia: J.P. Lippincott Co.

Prechtl, H.F.R. and Stemmer, J. (1962), Choreiform syndrome in children. *Developmental Medicine & Child Neurology*, 4:119-127.

_____(1978), Rapid silent response to repeated target symbols by dyslexic and non-dyslexic children. *Brain and Language*, 6:52-62.

Rapoport, J.L. (1978), Dextroamphetamine: cognitive and behavioral effects in normal prepubertal boys. *Science*, 199:560-563.

Ross, D. and Ross, S. (1976), *Hyperactivity: Research, Theory, and Action*. New York; John Wiley & Sons.

Rudel, R.G., Denckla, M.B. and Broman, M. (1978), Rapid silent response to repeated target symbols by dyslexic and non-dyslexic children. *Brain and Language*, 6:52-62.

Schain, R.J. (1975), Minimal brain dysfunction. *Current Problems in Pediatrics*, Vol. V., No. 10. Chicago: Year Book Medical Publishers, Inc.

Simpson, R.H. (1944), The specific meanings of certain terms indicating differing degrees of frequency. *Quarterly Journal of Speech*, 30:328-330.

Strauss, A.A. and Kephart, N.C. (1955), *Psychopathology and Education of the Brain-Injured Child*. Vol. II. New York: Grune & Stratton.

Strauss, A.A. and Lehtinen, L. (1947), *Psychopathology and Education of the Brain-Injured Child*, Vol. I. New York: Grune and Stratton.

Sykes, D., Douglas, V., and Morgenstern, G. (1972), The effect of methylphenidate on sustained attention in hyperactive children. *Psychopharmacologia* (Berl.), 5:262-274.

Terman, L. M. and Merrill, M. A. (1937), *Measuring Intelligence*, Boston: Houghton Mifflin.

_____ _____(1960), *Stanford-Binet Intelligence Scale*. Boston: Houghton-Mifflin Co.

Wechsler, D. (1974), *Wechsler Intelligence Scale for Children-Revised*. New York: The Psychological Corporation.

Wepman, J. M. (1973), *Auditory Discrimination Test*. Palm Springs, California: Language Research Associates.

Werry, J. S. (1968), Developmental hyperactivity. *Pediatric Clinics of North America*, 15:581-599.

Wyatt, G. (1969), *Language Learning and Communication Disorders in Children*. New York: Free Press.

Yaklovlev, P. and Lecours, A. (1967), The myelogenetic cycles of regional maturation of the brain. In: *Regional Development of the Brain in Early Life*, ed. A. Minkowski. Oxford and Edinburgh: Blackwell Scientific Publications.

Author Index

Subject Index